The Yapana® Way

Restorative Yoga Therapy
& the Art of Being

Leeann Carey

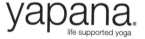

yapana.
life supported yoga

"Change is not something that we should fear. Rather, it is something that we should welcome. For without change, nothing in this world would ever grow or blossom, and no one in this world would ever move forward to become the person they're meant to be."

~ B. K. S. Iyengar

yapana.
life supported yoga

The Yapana Way

Restorative Yoga Therapy & the Art of Being

Leeann Carey

LeeannCareyYoga.com

ISBN-13:9780989733908
ISBN-10:0989733904

Photographer: Wendy Saade

Book Design: Wendy Saade

Cover Design: Genesis Moss

Editor: Ralph Cissne

CONTENTS

DEDICATION

I have been truly blessed with the opportunity to share yoga with gifted instructors, and to learn from master teachers, around the world. This book is dedicated to all of the yoga enthusiasts who have entrusted me with their process and the yoga teachers who have given their time, knowledge, and invaluable life lessons.

It is with sincere devotion I also offer a dedication to Kofi Busia (a.k.a. Boy Born on Friday), a devotee of yoga master B. K. S. Iyengar. I met Kofi in a Santa Monica workshop in the early 1990s. There began my interest and intention to share what yoga was trying to teach me. I often hear his voice, on and off the mat, telling me to stand upright, be steady throughout, and see things as they are.

Kofi's sharp communication skills, exceptional mind, and honest perspective about the yoga community and the teaching of yoga earned him a uniquely honored reputation among students and yoga teachers. No teacher has influenced me more in my practice, teaching, and perceptions of life – the ultimate practice of yoga.

For this, and so much more, I offer a special and wholehearted dedication to Kofi Busia, Boy Born on Friday.

With love and eternal gratitude,

Leeann

ACKNOWLEDGEMENTS

I extend special acknowledgement and gratitude to my family: Stephen, Robyn, Timothy, Alex, and Rob. For as long as I can remember, each one has supported me in my passion for yoga. I wish to acknowledge important people with whom I have developed business and personal relationships that have helped to make this book possible: Stephen Anderson, Jeff Homolya, Genesis Moss, Lisa Muehlenbein, Marc Newman, Wendy Saade, and Stacy Shimabukuro, and the book's models: The Carey kids, Yvette Hamara, Leilani Kashida, Jules Mitchell, Patrick Moore, Stacy Shimabukuro and Marla Landa Williams. Huge gratitude and thanks to each of you.

My heartfelt appreciation goes to my editor, Ralph Cissne. His insights and razor sharp attention to detail is without exception. I am grateful for the tireless effort he dedicated to seeing this project through, and for providing an organized and concise platform to be heard while remaining sensitive to my voice.

And to B. K. S. Iyengar, Kofi Busia, Donna Farhi, Judith Lasater, and Richard C. Miller, from whom I have received brilliant teachings on the art and science of yoga therapy. It is with utter gratitude and a humble heart that I stand on the shoulders of these teachers and so many more who have taught me so much.

I also wish to express special thanks to Wanda Marie, my spiritual sister, friend, mentor, and the greatest supporter of all I have ever tried or dreamed of doing.

Thank you, everyone.

I love you.

Yoga has been tested for thousands of years. It is more than an experiment or last resort. It is a proven path to wellness, healing, and longevity. It works.

INTRODUCTION

There are eight limbs (observances and restraints) of yoga that serve as guidelines. This book addresses the third limb, asana (posture or pose). Each of us experiences challenges and triumphs on the mat. Our challenges may present themselves in flexibility, mobility, stability, clarity, or in a host of other ways. I invite you to address the obstacles and opportunities you face on the mat with intelligence and a loving kindness. This book provides the tools and understanding to meet these challenges with a unique practice that teaches we are more than our bodies and more than what we do. This simple yet comprehensive guide will prompt an inquiry about the level of support required to meet yourself where you are, a process that evolves over time. We simply need to be there.

Yapana is an ancient Sanskrit word meaning, "The support and extension of life." Yapana Yoga Therapy is a physical practice that includes yoga props for strategic support to extend the life of poses, which supports and extends the nature of the experience. This style of yoga was developed based on decades of experience working with the physically challenged, professional athletes, yoga teachers and students just like you – those with an inquiring mind who want to deepen their practice and balance their ego.

Let's take a closer look.

This practice meets people where they are. It is designed to encourage self-inquiry, reflection and change, not perfection – the universe has already taken care of that part.

CHAPTER 1

YAPANA YOGA THERAPY

Yapana Yoga Therapy is a hatha yoga practice consisting of a series of simple movements to warm-up the body, followed by DOING (dynamic) and BEING (relaxing) poses held for an extended period of time with the support of yoga props, and ends with a STILL (final relaxation) pose to complete the practice.

This practice meets people where they are. It is designed to encourage self-inquiry, reflection and change, not perfection – the universe has already taken care of that part. It is a gateway to discover how to apply its therapeutic outcome on and off the mat. The objective on the mat is to promote both balance and a positive and enduring effect while supported in both the heat-building and passive phases of the practice.

For purposes of this book, the BEING and STILL segments of the practice are deconstructed and explored. Often times in a classical hatha yoga practice, yoga instructors and students value the stronger segment of the class more and as a result, do not give ample time for the rest and relaxation phases of the practice. Because we live in a fast-paced world, restorative poses are a necessary part of our practice to help restore us physically, mentally, emotionally, and spiritually. We all require recovery time, some more than others. If this part of our living is being incorporated into our yoga practice, it will take care of the stressors that may lie ahead.

BEING Poses (Supported Passive Poses)

BEING poses are the essential core of the Yapana practice. It is here where the body/mind is supported into a state of relaxation and recovery. BEING poses give the body an opportunity to stretch passively and the mind the opportunity to experience what comes from doing nothing while supported in a yoga pose to elicit body/mind relaxation.

BEING poses are unique in that they help to stimulate the parasympathetic nervous system, often referred to as the "rest and digest system," and is responsible for the stimulation of bodily functions that occur while at rest. Although the body is in "rest mode," this does not always mean that the mind will settle into a quiet place. As with all other styles of yoga, however, practice and patience are the doorways into stillness and the settling of the mind.

Strategic placement and the ample use of yoga props are crucial to encouraging a peaceful experience in the BEING poses. One of the roles of your bodily organs is to support the musculoskeletal system. The better the body is supported to meet you exactly where you are – stiff, flexible or with a wandering mind – the more fully the body/mind can relax. When all urges to "do" are relieved, the body/mind can surrender and relax into doing less and feeling more.

BEING poses are practiced in all categories of practice:

- Backbends
- Twists (seated, supine, and prone variations)
- Forward bends
- Inversions
- Miscellaneous (side lying, supine, and prone)

BEING poses are held with support anywhere from 2 to 20 minutes.
Refer to the Practice Time Table in Chapter 10.

STILL Pose (Savasana: Corpse Pose for Final Relaxation)

Savasana (Corpse Pose) is crucial to all styles of asana practices, but especially to complete a Yapana practice. Because BEING poses have prepared the body for final relaxation, to shorten or to all together ignore this part of the practice would leave the student feeling incomplete. Savasana is a pose for integrating all that has come before. When we stop planning, organizing, and managing, we are able – if only momentarily – to experience the death of our doing. When this occurs, the full experience of a present moment dying, is only a breath away. Death teaches us that time and space are temporary and that clinging to life is an aversion to change. Savasana acts as fertile ground that creates an opening for the passing and going of all that keeps us bound.

In a Yapana practice, we allow a minimum of 15 minutes for final relaxation. Studies show that within that time, many people can drop into a state of deep relaxation or what's considered the Alpha state of mind, in which time and space become irrelevant or rather nonexistent to your consciousness. Like in all yoga poses, there are levels of experience that change with time spent in a pose. It is not unlikely to be disturbed in Savasana, even after a complete practice. Disturbances can surface from physical, mental, or emotional agitations. Everyone responds differently to a practice, however, both thoughtful and skillful sequencing of the Yapana BEING and STILL segments will encourage the most amount of rest with the least amount of effort.

How Would You Like Your Savasana?

There are many ways to take rest in Savasana, with or without support. Savasana does not have to be practiced the exact same way every time. Determining the kind of Savasana for the practice is based on what kinds of poses, or Pranayama, were practiced before Savasana. For instance, if the sequence addressed a stiff lower back, it may be a logical choice to offer a Savasana that gives support to the lower back. If this is the case, consider practicing Savasana with either the legs elevated or weight on the top thighs to release the lower back into gravity. Or, if the sequence focused on opening the chest and shoulders, it may be a logical choice to offer a Savasana that includes an eye pillow to support going inside.

Preparation for a Pranayama (Breathing) Practice

Perhaps you offer a pranayama practice toward the end of the asana practice. If so, you may have taught poses that focus on opening the front, back and side waists, and the chest and shoulders. Practicing a "mini" Savasana (approximately 3 minutes) is recommended before a pranayama practice. This can help further mentally prepare for pranayama. Of course, after pranayama practice is completed, a full Savasana is recommended.

YOGA THERAPY – IT IS WHAT IT IS

Like so many others, I became interested in therapeutic yoga because at some point I experienced the value of an asana practice being more than a physical workout. Yoga therapy is the new buzz word in the yoga community, but what does it mean? After all, isn't all yoga considered therapeutic? Yes and no.

All yoga is therapeutic, whether it is passive or dynamic. What makes an intelligent yoga practice therapeutic is not one or the other, but whether or not it addresses the needs of the practitioners. Yoga therapy is not solely about practicing a relaxing yoga pose. It is about rightness: Using the right pose at the right time, in the right way for the right purpose. It fulfills an intention, purpose and direction. And it is a process and road map for discovering what works for YOU while giving you the tools to integrate a vigilant understanding of how you do life on and off the mat.

After all, yoga (yug = to yolk, unite) is trying to teach us that it is not just about "me" (the ego) or what I'm trying to achieve (the pose, breathing practice, life skill, etc.). It is about joining the two in a way that is mindful, meaningful, and extends well beyond the yoga mat. Simply stated, therapeutic yoga is about skillfully reconciling differences specific to your needs, while drawing from the rooftop of your awareness to what is happening, while it is happening.

OVERVIEW – WHY USE YOGA PROPS?

B. K. S. Iyengar introduced props into the modern practice of yoga to allow all practitioners access to the benefits of the postures regardless of physical condition, age, or length of study. The central purpose for using yoga props is to address a need for support. Some people like to rename yoga props to sound more appealing, like yoga "toys" or "tools." I am not opposed to doing this, although personally I've never found the need. A "prop" is just that. It is supportive and helpful when facing obstacles on the mat because it helps to meet us where we are. That's the job it is intended to do. A prop is a prop. No amount of calling it something other than it is will change the purpose. What will change is the understanding and popularity with intelligent, creative, and confident use.

Props help practitioners at all levels gain the sensitivity of a pose while receiving the benefits over time without overextending yourself. It allows students to practice asanas (postures) and pranayama (breath control) with greater effectiveness, ease, and stability. Still and yet, some may be resistant to receiving support from yoga props because it is a pointer back to themselves. But isn't most everything? If you assign a negative attitude toward prop support you may feel as though you are "cheating" in your practice and may generally oppose support in other areas of your life. Or perhaps requiring additional support shines a light on a shadow that you would prefer not to address. This I know for sure, if yoga instructors do not value using props their students won't either. My experience over decades of teaching is that those instructors only lack the skill of how to intelligently and creatively use them. I wrote this book to help students and educate yoga instructors how to use yoga props, demystify them, and inspire yoga enthusiasts everywhere to play and soften their edges on the mat with strategic and creative prop support.

We're ready to move forward.

WHO BENEFITS?

Don't believe anyone who says using yoga props on the mat is cheating. One of my yoga teachers taught that asana practice is more about subtraction than addition (thank you, Richard C. Miller), and using yoga props can help every sincere student to drop into that understanding.

It's perfectly fine to practice without the support of yoga props. It's just that in all the years I have shared yoga with different people at different levels of practice, I have yet to find one person, not one, that didn't benefit from using a yoga prop in one or more yoga poses. From the most flexible and strong, to the least, a strategically placed yoga prop can elevate the physical and spiritual trajectory of your yoga practice.

In case you're not sure, I've highlighted how prop support can benefit yoga practitioners. Perhaps you'll recognize yourself in one of the groups below.

Yoga Newbies

If you are new to yoga, this book will help ease your way into the restorative journey. It will prepare you for practicing in a full-service yoga studio where use of yoga props is commonplace. As a beginning student there is so much to learn. Prop support encourages students to investigate and organize themselves mindfully, rather than imposing hard and fast rules of destination and time. This kind of learning fosters patience, acceptance and self-reflection. These are the cornerstones of a mindful practice and one that has legs to grow for a lifetime.

Yoga Enthusiasts

Let's say you're a yoga practitioner that practices a minimum of once or twice a week. Whether you are currently using yoga props or not, this book will help to refine your practice and develop your "inner" teacher. This book will help you to play your physical and mental edges in a thoughtful way and can even inspire you to begin a home practice. Start by working with your favorite yoga pose, one that feels comfortable to you. Next, determine how long you can stay in the pose maintaining that level of comfort. Once discomfort surfaces, take note of the part of you that begins to tire. Feel your way into what's happening and identify your greatest sensations.

Now try coming into the pose with prop support that allows you to maintain the pose a little longer, perhaps extending it's comfort and shelf life for twice the time you had originally practiced the pose without support. Play around with the support until you are certain that it provides a level of experience that allows you to breathe smoothly, maintain safe alignment skills, and a calm mind. Part of developing your "inner teacher" is to have a curiosity about what's happening "now," and to listen and follow your intuition. Your body/mind is brilliant. Your practice will speak to you in both quiet and loud voices. You only need to observe, listen, adjust and wait. You'll be exercising the mind of your inner yoga teacher, an invaluable tool whether practicing by yourself or in a group class.

Yoga Teachers

Being of service through yoga is a rewarding experience. As an ambassador for yoga, you have signed up to practice, continue your studies and spread the heart of yoga with others. This book will teach you how to see and teach your students, not just lead poses. Learning how to intelligently, skillfully, and creatively advise and adjust your students with prop support will enhance the overall quality of your teaching and their practice. Many students fail to discover the benefits of passive restorative yoga because their teacher may not be trained in that style. Learning how to use yoga props will open your students to experience a whole and balanced practice. A teacher that values the restorative side of yoga understands what lies beneath what's so obvious in a practice – that timing is valued over timeliness and process is valued over progress. These are the just some of the rich lessons I have learned from my teachers.

You too, can be this kind of teacher. The more you educate yourself on how to work individually with your students, the more yoga they will experience and the less ego they will fuel. Observing your students without yoga prop support paints a picture of where they can build and let go. Using yoga props to guide your students is a path to work within their limitations and safely maximize the benefits of the pose. This style of teaching clears the way for reconciling differences – yoga's ultimate path to freedom.

Weekend Warriors and Professional Athletes

More and more sport enthusiasts and professional athletes are integrating yoga into their fitness routine. Weekend warriors and professional athletes require considerable active recovery to balance the effects of intense workouts. Unfortunately, a quieter practice is not always welcomed. What is required is a slowing down from sweating and endorphin chasing, but also a kind of mind that seeks stillness from doing nothing but feeling and breathing. It's difficult for most of us, but promising for all.

The BEING poses are particularly helpful to stretch, lengthen and open areas that are typically overworked. A yoga practice that includes BEING poses promotes flexibility, an important equation of injury prevention. Flexibility helps you to tap into your strength. Strength and flexibility go hand in hand. One without the other is like a table missing a leg – simply out of balance. In addition, a pranayama practice is an extremely helpful tool that fosters a stable, calm and present state of mind, and can translate into improving your athletic performance and sharpening your ability to focus.

Injury Management

An intelligent yoga practice can address a host of physical, emotional and spiritual concerns. Ancient yoga philosophy states that each of us is made of five koshas (sheaths): physical, energy (breath or life force), mind (intellect), perception (intuition, wisdom) and spiritual (innate joy, peace and harmony). My yoga practice has proven to me that these layers are connected much like the anklebone is connected to the hipbone. Although the two bones may not be close in proximity, if one is affected the other may likely be. Since yoga therapists are not doctors, it can be a risk to treat any chronic condition with certainty, however, it is wise to apply yogic principles and therapies that have proven successful, using a basic tried and true balanced approach including most or all of the following:

- Relaxation
- Traction (if there is compression)
- Mobility
- Stability and Strength
- Flexibility

For decades I have used this simple recipe with yoga students to help them manage and recover from injuries. It doesn't mean that students with severe issues avoided necessary surgery. However, I have prescribed many yoga recipes using this approach, which can include both DOING and BEING poses, or one or the other, all practiced with yoga prop support to prepare students for pre-surgery and speed up the recovery time post surgery. Again, I can't stress enough how important it is to link all "layers" for holistic healing and productive injury management.

Massage Therapists

If you are a massage therapist, you may already be stretching your clients. In my opinion, integrating massage with a few targeted BEING poses that address your clients' habitual holding patterns is a hot house for deep letting go. It is a unique experience to be supported in a passive yoga pose by both gravity and strategically placed yoga props. It always encourages a deep level of relaxation that may otherwise be difficult to access through assisted stretching. Here there is nothing to do and nowhere to go. Your clients can be suspended in the experience of a yoga prop-supported stretch while breathing, feeling, sensing and letting go. Sounds good, right?

That which I seek finds me, embraces me and knows me.
It lives inside me.

CHAPTER 2
MEET YOUR YOGA PROPS

Each of the yoga props listed (except for the eye pillow) can be practiced in all classifications of yoga poses – standing, seated, back bending, twisting, inverting and forward
bending – whether they are DOING or BEING poses. I have my personal prop preferences
in style, size, material, and manufacturer. For the budget-minded yogi, however, don't let
the expense of yoga props deter you from creating an ample prop inventory. When I first
started teaching I used books for blocks, towels for blankets, couch pillows for bolsters,
dining room chairs, fabric remnants sewed together for belts (trust me, I am NOT a seam-
stress!), and a kitchen sink and door jams for leverage (yes, even a kitchen sink!). All is
possible. All the time. Always. Think outside the box.

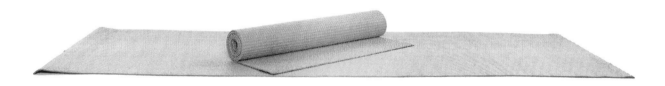

Yoga Mat

Yoga mat manufacturers produce mats in various thicknesses. For ample support, whether
the mat requires folding or rolling, it should measure no more than 3/16-inch deep, and
I prefer a non-skid mat for sufficient stickiness. This guarantees the holding in place of
other yoga props that may be used in combination with the mat. Check out local yoga
studios that may be replacing old mats. You might be able to purchase a used mat for a
buck or two. Just clean the you-know-what out of them and use them for props. Consider

reaching out to your yoga buddies and find out if anyone has an extra mat they no longer use because they didn't like it. The plethora of mats I've collected over the years include expensive mats people have purchased, but didn't like for one reason or another. If I can't use the entire mat as a prop, I cut them up into various-sized square sheets and use them as pads for boney body parts and lifts for feet. Get creative!

How to use: Yoga mats can be used for cushioning boney body parts, holding blocks, blankets, bolsters and chairs in place or rolled up into tubes as a substitute for blankets or bolsters. The best yoga mats are quite sticky, can easily roll and are no thicker than 3/16-inch. The wonderful thick mats that are now on the market are great for lying and practicing, but they are often far too thick to use as a prop.

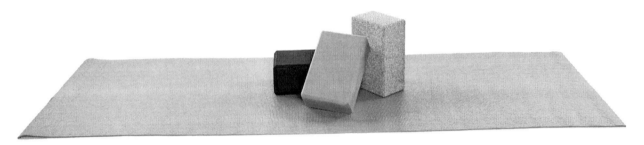

Blocks

A cork block is my preference due to its unique combination of stability, weight and movability to slide against the floor when necessary. Practitioners may prefer foam blocks, which are easy to carry because of their lightweight material and the level of cushion they provide. I like foam blocks for cushion, but they are not stable, therefore, I don't recommend them for supporting standing poses or some backbends. Yoga blocks come in all sizes. I like the standard size, which is 4" x 6" x 9". It is convenient, however, to have a few different sizes. Sometimes a student needs a 4" x 6" x 9" block and another block half that dimension. If you don't have a block, consider using a book, preferably one you've already read so you don't get distracted.

How to use: Blocks can be used to bring the floor to you to assist with flexibility or to wake up dull areas of your body. They also help to "reduce the reach," access core stability, and provide unique leverage in far reaching forward bends. Blocks are very versatile and you will love them.

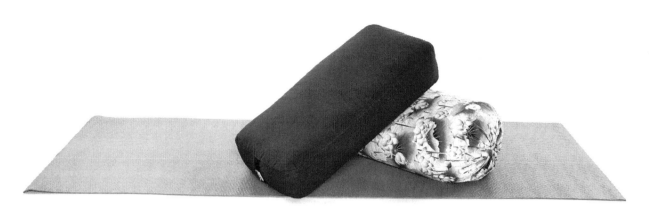

Bolster

Bolsters come in all sizes and shapes. Finding the right-sized bolster for you is important. If you are petite like me, a bolster that is half your body size doesn't always work. Too much support isn't helpful and not enough defeats the purpose. I recommend you begin with a standard size bolster. You can always add folded blankets on top to create more height when needed. The most commonly used bolster is a standard "flat" bolster, measuring 8" x 27" x 32.5" that weighs 5 lbs. An oval bolster, measuring 9" x 26" x 34.5" weighs 7 lbs. Choosing the right bolster for each pose and each person depends on the level of support needed in relation to your unique needs and how it best supports the trajectory of the pose.

How to use: One word, YES! Bolsters do just that – they bolster a part of the body in order to open, release, or support that part. They are truly a godsend.

Wall

Use a clean, sturdy and flat wall without glass or a mirror. Besides using a chair, a wall is my favorite yoga prop. You can push against, relax into, leverage from and confront your fears with its support. Everyone has a wall in their house, yoga studio or gym. They may, however, have mirrors attached to them. Do not use a mirrored wall, but if that's all you have proceed with caution. I don't recommend flipping up into a handstand on a mirrored wall unless you are certain of it's stability and security. When using a chair against a mirrored wall, simply pad the back rest of the chair with a blanket to prevent scratching or breaking the mirror. In a pinch, you can use a securely closed door with a flat surface. Also, the corner of where two walls meet provide excellent alignment feedback of either side of the body. Try it and notice what you feel.

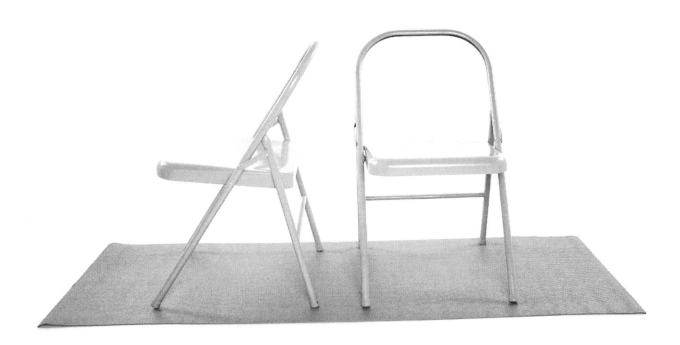

Chair or Stool

A sturdy folding chair with the reinforcement bar in the back and the back rest of the chair pushed out. If you hammer out the chair back rest, be sure to file any rough edges. Another option is to wrap the back of the frame with athletic tape. I learned that nifty trick from one of the LCY mentors and it works well because it also offers a nice grip for your hands. I learned my lesson working with athletes up to 6' 9". The standard folding chair is too short (Thanks, Luke!). In this case, it might be best in some yoga poses to use a stool, or prop your chair on blocks to make it taller. If you are working in a gym environment, I like stacking aerobic steps because they provide a stable seat that sometimes a stool does not. And, there is a new folding chair on the market that extends the normal height up to six inches. There isn't an excuse not to use one.

How to use: The chair is another favorite yoga prop of mine as it can provide a little more "restful" support. When necessary, you can drop all of your body weight into the seat surface. I've included some very creative approaches to poses with the support of a chair. Note, sometimes you need to position the chair next to a wall so that it doesn't move.

Blankets

Be particular about your blankets. The ones made entirely out of polyester are difficult to fold and those that are strictly wool generate a funky smell after continued use and care. What to do? Purchase blankets that are a mix of the two materials. If you want to avoid the expense, use what you can afford and is readily available. Even folded up blankets from your house, bath or beach towels will work. Use what works for you and provides the level of support needed.

How to use: Blankets can be used to bring the floor to you, cushion hard areas, and weight down an area of the body to help it release. If you don't have bolsters you can fold blankets and stack them into the shape of a bolster. Rolled or folded, they provide excellent support for chest openers, twists and forward bends. Some BEING poses will require short or long-rolled blankets, while other times a double or accordion-folded blankets. No matter which shape you use, always roll and fold the blankets so they have clean edges as they are supporting your body weight. Blankets fall apart when they are not carefully shaped and this will effect the level of support they are intended to provide.

Many folds and rolls begin with the Single-Folded blanket called Foundation. From this shape you can make just about any of the required shapes.

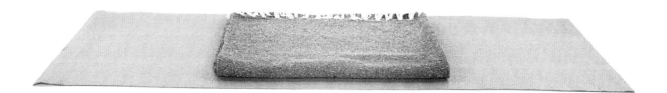

How to fold a Single-Folded blanket – FOUNDATION
1. Starting with the short ends of a blanket, fold it in half.
2. From the short ends, fold it in half again two more times.
3. Smooth out any wrinkles and straighten the edges.

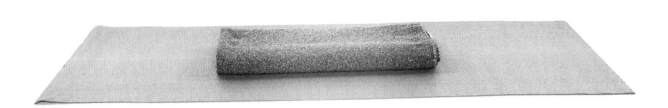

How to fold a Double-Folded blanket

1. Start with a Foundation blanket shape.
2. Fold it in half from the long, clean edges.
3. Smooth out any wrinkles and straighten the edges.

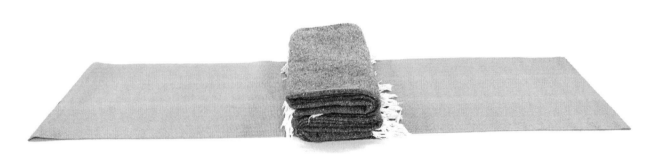

How to fold Two-Double Folded Stacked blankets (as a Bolster)

1. Stack two double-folded blankets so that the clean and open edges are aligned.
2. Smooth out any wrinkles and straighten the edges.

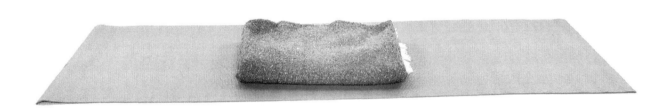

How to fold a Meditation Pad blanket

1. Start with a Foundation blanket shape.
2. From the short clean edge, fold in half.
3. Smooth out any wrinkles and straighten the edges.

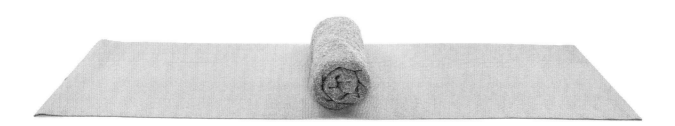

How to roll a Short-Rolled blanket

1. Start with a Foundation blanket shape.
2. From the long clean edge, tightly roll into a solid cylinder.
3. Smooth out any wrinkles and straighten the edges.

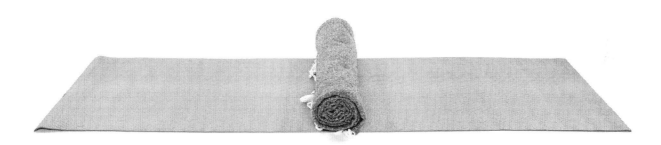

How to roll a Long-Rolled blanket

1. Start with a Foundation blanket shape.
2. From the short clean edge, tightly roll into a solid cylinder.
3. Smooth out any wrinkles and straighten the edges.

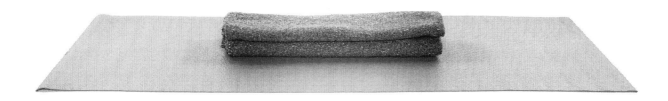

How to fold an Accordion-Folded blanket

1. Start with a Foundation blanket shape.
2. From the long clean edge, fold in quarters accordion style.
3. Smooth out any wrinkles and straighten the edges.

Belt

Belts also come in many sizes. I prefer using 10' belts because they provide the most options. It's better to have a longer belt than a shorter one. That way you avoid tieing belts together to make a long one. That's confusing. The difference in price of a 6' belt and a 10' belt is insignificant compared to the benefits of working with a longer one. I also recommend the D-ring belts as they provide the best locking system and are easiest to adjust. Yes, the D-ring belt is my favorite, but you can make a similar prop by sewing fabric. I encourage you to invest in a real yoga belt. When you do, you won't be sorry.

How to use: Belts stabilize joints, encourage flexibility, support inflexibility and create traction and space – two magic words in yoga therapy, as many suffer compression somewhere. Using a yoga belt can provide instant relief for some people. Need I say more?

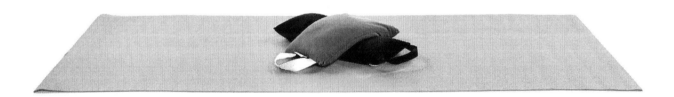

Sandbag

The sandbag is another genius idea from B. K. S. Iyengar. It's a yoga prop that provides weight and encourages release to overworked areas. Yapana therapy students are hooked on sandbags. Classical weight plates were once used, the old-school kind that are still used in gyms. Imagine being in Savasana (Corpse Pose) with a few large round weights stacked on top of the pelvis and legs? Don't laugh until you try it. I'll try just about anything that I think might provide the kind of support I might need at any given time. Or you can make your own sandbags. Whether you use sand (don't steal it from the beach, buy it from the store), pea gravel, rice, or some other content for the bag, be sure that you do not fill the bag to the rim as this prevents you from adjusting the bag to work with it in segments when needed. It needs to be malleable so you can manipulate it to rest partially on a limb if needed.

Do This:

1. When placing the bags at the top thighs in a supine BEING pose, be sure the knees are either on the same plane as the hips or no more than one inch above.

2. When grounding the low back, place the bag directly across the back in a horizontal position with the short ends of the bag facing each hip.

3. Any time you use the bag to ground the shoulders in a supine BEING pose, the back of the shoulder should not be more than an inch off the ground.

Don't Do This:

1. Never place the bag directly on the knee joints when they are in a flexed lateral position.

2. Never place the bags directly on the knees unless you are following a specific therapeutic practice that you know well for a specific purpose, which will encourage a specific result that you specifically understand. The weight of a sandbag on the knees in some straight legged seated positions with additional prop support can help to stretch tight ligaments. But you must know what, how and why you are doing this. People will place a 10 lb. sandbag just about anywhere thinking it will help. This will not help when used unwiselessly.

In general, be mindful of how and why you use sand bags around joints.

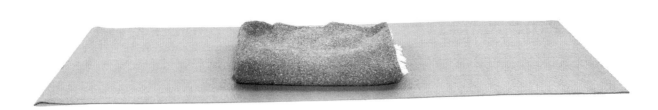

Meditation Pad/Zafu

A meditation pad supports the spine to lift while in a seated position. Some practitioners use "zafu," a Japanese word for "round cushion." Will your meditation be better while sitting on a zafu? That depends. My first mediation teacher taught me how to calm my mind on a street bench while traffic was bustling around me. Would sitting on a zafu have made it better? I have no idea. For some people, however, it's more about assigning a feeling or discipline to the object, kind of like a yoga mat. Can we have an active asana (posture) practice without a mat? Absolutely. Do we care for our yoga mats like they are real estate? Some of us do. In the end, the true value of having a meditation zafu or meditation pad made from folding a blanket, is that it lifts the pelvis from the legs, which makes sitting upright easier.

How to use: Sit on it and practice being still. That's it.

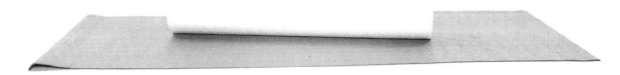

Foam Roller

Two words: Love it! Foam rollers come in all sizes and levels of density and help to massage large muscles groups and fascia, the fibrous cartilage which covers the muscles. It's almost like getting a massage except you don't have to pay for it, remove your clothes or get greased with oil. It does a great job of breaking up lactic acid and you're in control of the pressure and duration. Of course, rolling on a tennis ball also does the trick, but the body rollers are far superior. Sometimes I like to start a class, private session or my own practice with the foam roller to encourage oxygen and blood flow to muscles. Other times I might end with the roller. It all depends on what I'm trying to support in the practice.

How to use: Just roll your body across it. You can roll across the front, back and side body. Roll slowly. If you rip through it at lightening speed you won't feel or realize its effects.

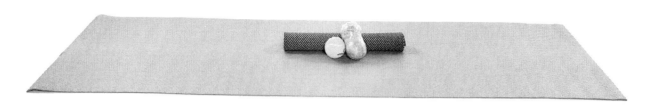

Tennis Ball

As mentioned above, if you don't have a foam roller, a tennis ball can be an adequate and inexpensive replacement. What's nice about using tennis balls is that they can target the small muscles groups to really get in there and work.

How to use: Roll the soles of your feet against it – wonderful for those suffering from plantar fascittus, a symptom caused from tight sole foot tendons. Basically, use it like the foam roller, but since the surface isn't nearly as large, be careful about pushing up against the spinal column. Just roll on either side of the spine. You can also tape two tennis balls together so each ball can roll up and down each side of the spinal column simultaneously.

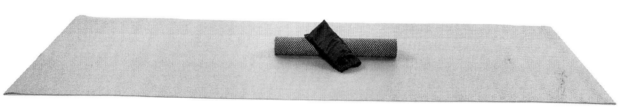

Eye Pillow

This is sort of like Goldilocks and The Three Bears. You may like an eye pillow that also covers the entire forehead. Or perhaps you want one that only covers the eye lids and bridge of the nose or somewhere in between. Why not have a combination of all so you can use them accordingly? If you are handy with a sewing machine you can make these yourself. If you do, please be sure to make a removable and washable cover to avoid eye infections from accumulated dirt, dust and use.

How to use: I consider eye pillows wonderful little gifts from yoga heaven. They can be used to block out the light, give a little bit of weight to the forehead, inside the palm of your hands or provide a cool support against the back of your neck. They support a meaningful turning inward.

GOING DEEPER

....

THE RIGHTNESS OF PRACTICE

....

Much of an intelligent and creative yoga practice is getting yourself to see the wisdom of why and what you are doing. It is up to you to bring the kind of awareness to your practice that clarifies that you choose for your practice to be meaningful. You will never know what comes from your practice if you don't practice with devotion, concentration, and faith.

Learning a Skill

The right prop support can teach a skill necessary for experiencing a balanced approach for doing, being and breathing in a yoga pose. Some solutions for addressing difficulties in a pose may often be found in other poses that require less. And they will always include a soft breath and a calm mind. In essence, a yielding body and mind. Yoga poses not only require strength, stability, flexibility and mobility, but also skills such as proprioception (1), somatic movement (2) and a mind that doesn't react to its fluctuations. If one or more of these skills are significantly impaired, the benefits are that much harder to access. For instance, let's use a simple backbend as an example.

Backbends require the chest muscles to stretch, mid/upper back muscles to contract, shoulder mobility, and the fibrous tissue between the mid/upper back vertebra to move forward. Muscles that are too tight and joints that are too stiff end up relying on help from other areas of the body that aren't meant to play a significant role in the pose. In a classic backbending pose, this can put strain on the lower segment of the spine and disrupt proper rotation of the shoulder joints. These imbalances, if not addressed, make it difficult to open and lift the chest with strong back body support, a skill necessary for a safe backbend. Therefore, safe and enjoyable backbends are often inaccessible to many students.

(1) Proprioception: The unconscious perception of movement and spatial orientation arising from stimuli within the body itself.

(2) Somatic movement: Movement that relies on your awareness, desire, and ability to become more self-determining. Somatic refers to your ability to sense the processes going on "within" you.

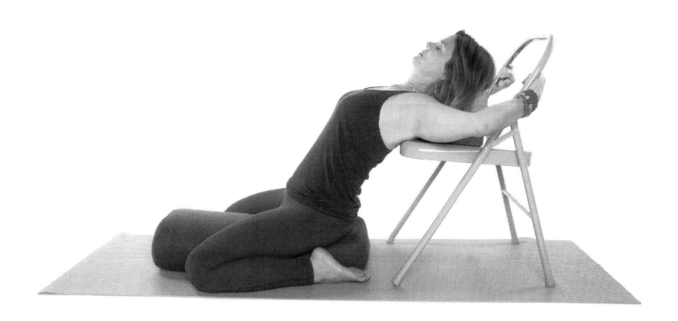

This photo demonstrates a simple chair supported Ustrasana (Camel Pose). This variation allows you to breathe and soften in the pose, and explore areas that otherwise would not safely be available in a backbend. Here you can investigate the skill necessary without additional load on the low back, while stretching and contracting the muscles needed to support a healthy backbend. Benefits abound.

Acceptance – Meeting Yourself Where You Are

I am reminded of a workshop I taught for yoga teachers at a body/mind conference. We covered a lot of pose breakdowns, which is always rewarding. Troubleshooting solutions for different body types is a little like being in a lab. You never know how one insight will lead to another, so it is important to be open to the process. The only formula I know for this is meeting students where they are. I practice this acceptance on the mat. It's not always easy, but it is always inspiring.

Throughout my travels, I've had the privilege of working with yoga instructors and students from all over North America and Canada. My experience in general is that too many practitioners feel badly when they run across a yoga pose they cannot execute well. What's worse, I have perceived embarrassment and almost shame. I hear rumblings like, "My shoulders aren't as flexible as Eric's." Or teachers share their concern when they aren't as mobile as some of their students. My advice. Welcome acceptance.

NEWS FLASH: There may be poses that you will never be able to practice well without accepting additional support. Or you may come to the realization that some poses aren't right for your body type. Don't feel defeated. Instead, consider this as a giving moment to embrace what is present. Adjust to the utter kindness of accepting support and letting go into what's happening now. Strategic yoga prop support can help you learn how to safely and efficiently leverage your strengths, play with weaknesses, and explore them with a soft breath and calm mind. Sweet relief.

When you step on your mat do you ask, "How can I grow today?" or "How can I be more of myself today?" The time on our mat can be used to address these deep questions by recognizing and attending to our individual needs at the moment. Meeting ourselves where we are shines a light on what may be a missing ingredient in many yoga practices: acceptance and mindfulness of what is happening now. Learning how to efficiently use the body and breath as resources to focus, grow or transform, can bring attention to opening and integrating the Light that lives within.

I have a history of tight hamstrings, calves, and a tight mid/upper back. This makes forward bends of all kinds my least favorite poses.

This variation of Paschimottanasana (Seated Forward Bend Pose) offers the kind of support needed to move gently into the stretch of my tight legs and back. Yes, it's a lot of support, but I'm not too proud to accept it. Over the years of practicing this variation from time to time, it has helped me to make great leaps in my forward bending. It has improved my flexibility and, more importantly, it has taught me how to be more patient in a pose that I previously considered to be my nemesis.

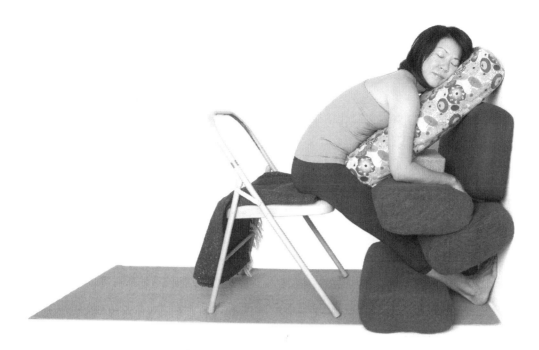

Make It Calmer

Support also comes in the form of feeling that you are so well taken care of that you can completely surrender. Ahhh – nothing quite like it. The body and mind may require a level of healing in a yoga pose that can only be offered when properly supported.

Tom has had a couple of bad bouts with his low back giving out. One evening he walked into my house for a casual dinner party I was hosting for friends. I watched him walk with a strong lean to one side, like a crab walking on the ocean's uneven sandy bottom. After a visit to the doctor and some yoga therapy, his back healed. But there's nothing more satisfying to someone who has been dealing with back pain to voice an audible "ahhh" when put into a supported yoga pose that provides both physical release and mental relief.

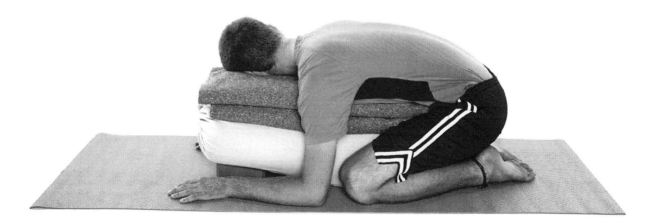

A well supported Balasana (Child Pose). Just what the doctor ordered.

STRATEGIC PROP PLACEMENT

Pose Alignment and Misalignment

Much of the time we don't know what we are doing while we are doing it, even on the yoga mat. All kinds of misalignments occur without awareness because habits have deep roots that are invisible to us – that's why they are called habits. Yoga props help you highlight those common and repeated misalignments by preventing us from overworking mobile areas, or stabilizing and stretching underworked ones.

Bring the Pose to You

This is an important element to having a safe and effective Yapana practice. If the prop support is inaccurate and does not meet your needs, the benefits of the pose are compromised. There are two ways to bring the pose to you, either by reducing the reach or broadening the base. Each of these address our flexibility and/or mobility challenges. And they take strain away from the joints and unnecessary load to one or more segments of the spine. Both should encourage space and traction, or extension and contraction when required.

Awakening Consciousness

A yoga prop can awaken dormant areas of the body, thereby, stimulating a part of the pose that was previously unreachable. If the only reason a part of a pose has been avoided is due to inflexibility, the right prop support will build awareness to an unvisited area and create a pathway to improved flexibility.

Quieting Overworked Areas

It's common to overdue yoga poses. Props help all practitioners (including the most advanced) gain sensitivity by turning off the larger muscles groups and turning on the smaller ones. Yoga props provide support for the overworked areas of the body, allow the mind to relax, and more profoundly receive the benefits of the practice.

Whether you seek to awaken consciousness or quiet overworked areas, props provide feedback to make adjustments in both the body and the mind.

Sweet Sensation

There's nothing wrong with a prop supported yoga pose that just makes you feel, "Ahhh." In fact, this is the start of getting in touch with the "rest and digest" system at the center of this practice and the goal in all of the BEING poses.

Wait

You may set yourself up in a prop-supported pose and not feel the level of stretch you typically feel when practiced without support. This happens. What you need to know is sometimes you have to let the pose "bake" for a while. You have to wait. When a pose is well supported, different than being too supported, you may not feel anything because you are used to the immediate feedback you receive from larger muscle groups firing. Give yourself a bit of time, perhaps a minute or so, to allow the smaller muscles to begin to fire and the sensations begin to percolate. Based on your experience you can adjust accordingly.

Over Propped is Overrated

Be careful not to over-prop the poses. Recognize the architecture and trajectory of the pose to maintain safe alignment skills and intelligent support that promotes a smooth and steady breath, and a calm mind. The body should be able to move, if necessary, while in the pose. Notice if the body is moving in relation to the breath – is it concentrated in one area, or is no movement present? Too many props result in falling into or pushing away from the support. There is a better way.

Pose Trajectory – What Are You Trying to Achieve?

Each pose has a certain architecture, which supports the classification of the pose whether it is standing, back bending, twisting, forward bending, side bending, sitting or inverting. They all have an intention, purpose and direction and offer different remedies for the body and mind. Maintaining the trajectory of the pose when supporting it will help you achieve why you are practicing it. For instance, if the BEING backbend that you have propped is not bending the back, clearly, it can no longer be considered a backbend. That's why sometimes you have to give up something in order to get something else. Read on.

Give Up Something to Get Something Else

You may find that some of the poses don't work for your level of flexibility – DON'T WORRY. What is unique about Yapana practice is that you can attend to those inflexible areas by permitting yourself to safely target them even if you have to give up some of the pose. Ask yourself:

Why are you practicing a forward bend? So you can stretch your hamstrings, soothe and calm your central nervous system, or both? If you are pushing yourself in the pose due to tight hamstrings and it doesn't lend a smooth and steady breath and calm mind, it's not going to calm the nervous system.

Which is most important to you right now? Does stretching your hamstrings have precedence over the cooling effects of a forward bend or vice versa? Either answer is acceptable and valuable. If you need to address your hamstrings, give up the forward bend and safely target the hamstrings in another supported pose that doesn't require you to do a forward bend. If you need to calm your central nervous system, consider practicing a pose that calms your nervous system and doesn't pull on short hamstrings. Yapana practice can answer what you want and how you can approach it, while being supported throughout the journey.

Help for Hyperextension

A hyperextended joint is one that moves well beyond its natural range of motion. As a result, it places additional strain on ligaments and tendons, which help to prevent excessive motion. When these tissues are too loose, the joint is insecure and can result in injury. Hyperextension also creates misalignment and poor movement habits that can set the state for arthritis and other serious injuries. A strategically placed yoga prop can teach how to access neighboring muscles needed to prevent further damage.

Hyperextended Knees

In normal standing alignment, the leg forms a straight line from ankle to hip, with knees over ankles and hips over knees. If the knee is hyperextended, however, the legs will appear to curve back with the knees behind an imaginary straight line drawn from ankles to hips. One leg may hyperextend more than the other. Yoga poses cannot shorten over-stretched knee ligaments, but choosing the right poses with the proper support can help stabilize the knees by strengthening the neighboring muscles.

Those who hyperextend their knee have difficulty straightening their legs without over-stretching. Because none of the BEING poses require standing, there is less impact on the joints. There are, however, some BEING poses that require straight and firm legs, like seated forward bends. These poses can over-stretch the knee ligaments unless they are properly supported. One rule of thumb is to support the backs of the knees with minimal support. The support acts as a dam and prevents the knees from moving too far back so it doesn't load the weight into ligamentous tissue. This will be especially helpful in protecting the knees in forward bends. When the torso moves forward, it uses gravity as leverage and introduces force to the legs and spine.

Adding, Reducing, or Filling Space

A BEING pose may require more prop height (adding space) due to a lack of flexibility in order to avoid being stiff in the pose. Other times a pose will require more prop height (adding space) due to hyper mobility in order to avoid falling or collapsing.

A BEING pose may require less height (reducing space) due to general flexibility in order to avoid being too propped in the pose by the height of a bolster or block.

A BEING pose may require empty space be filled between the support, a limb or body part, and the floor so that the body doesn't feel as though it is in pieces. Or, so that the distal (furthest away) part of the limb is not hanging off the largest joint. Use support to fill the spaces between a student's body and the floor so that the body can receive feedback from the support. This helps to bring the floor to the student and prevents falling or rigidity in the pose.

Things to watch:

- Sharp angles in the body – The lines of the body should be round and soft, especially in the spine. If you see the lumbar (lower back) extended and the thorax (middle back) flat in a backbend (like an L shape) this is indicative that all the segments of the spine are not getting equal work and the load of the pose is resting in the lumbar. Ouch!

- Place, replace and adjust props to support the body so that all angles are soft.

- Use enough props so the pose "energy flow" is not falling backward or behind the head in a Backbend.

- Collapsing downward in the mid-torso in a Forward Bend.

- Collecting in the neck in a Twist.

- Falling behind the head or collapsing in the lumbar spine in an Inversion.

SAFE ALIGNMENT SKILLS (SAS) FOR BEING POSES

All movement requires that alignment principles are maintained in order to avoid injuries, and the practice of BEING poses is no exception to that rule. These important skills must be maintained in all BEING poses.

Foundation

The foundation of any pose is where everything starts. Perhaps you have heard the foundation of a yoga pose being compared to the foundation of a house. It's true. If the foundation of the pose is poor it affects the rest of the posture. In BEING poses, the set-up of the pose provides a solid foundation for safely and easily being and breathing in the pose. No exceptions.

- The body should be positioned with safe and secure alignment.

- The yoga props should be supportive providing both opportunities for stability and flexibility.

Pelvic Positions

There are three pelvic positions.

1. **Neutral:** Pelvis level with natural curve in the lumbar (lower spine).

2. **Anterior Tilt:** Pelvis tilts forward bringing the tailbone up and back and the pubis forward.

3. **Posterior Tilt:** Pelvis tilts back bringing the tailbone under and the pubis up.

In any given BEING pose, depending upon the architecture, one of above positions may be required. Generally, a backbend will require a posterior tiled pelvis, a forward bend will require an anterior tilted pelvis, and inversions, twists, and poses that are practiced supine or prone require a neutral pelvis.

Hip Hinge

Many people bend at the hips and waist at the same time when moving forward from an upright (standing or seated) position. Such biomechanics create a considerable strain on the lumbar. When bending forward either from a standing or seated position, we want to encourage bending at the hips while maintaining a neutral spine and pelvis. A proper Hip Hinge is necessary in all forward bending, and requires two-thirds extension into the pose prior to flexion.

Shoulder Stability/Mobility

The shoulder is a very complicated part of the human body. It is entirely dependent on non-boney connections for integrity. Yoga poses that help to create both stability and free up mobility are key to injury prevention and good posture. Healthy function of the shoulder is a delicate balance of strength, flexibility, core stability and alignment. Some asanas require shoulder stability while others require more mobility.

Shoulder Mobility

There are day-to-day activities that keep the head in a forward position that forces the shoulders to be rounded and the chest to sink. From sitting for long hours at the computer to driving in the car, over time, this poor postural habit will reduce shoulder mobility (the ability to have free range of motion in the shoulder) and, as a result, develop chronic tension in the neck and upper back. Some BEING poses require shoulder mobility. Safe alignment is paramount to maintain shoulder mobility. Follow these simple rules:

- Drop the shoulders away from the ears.

- When stretching the arms overhead, draw the upper arm bones into the shoulder sockets and keep the shoulder blades firm against the back. This will stabilize the shoulders and enhance movement of upper extremity when the shoulders goes through its ranges of motion.

Lighten the Load

There are times when you may need to "lighten the load" in any one of the BEING poses in order to transfer weight equally through the position and maintain SAS. The following are two ways to lighten the load:

Broaden the Base

Broadening the base is needed when more space is required to better access flexibility and SAS. For instance, in Paschimottanasana (Seated Forward Bend Pose), you might require more room in your hips in order to manage short hamstrings, which tend to pull the pelvis under in this seated position. Widening the legs a bit can give more space to the hips and that also will help with the Hip Hinge SAS.

Reduce the Reach

Reducing the reach of a pose, whether it is in the lower or upper body, helps to bring the pose to the student rather than the student to the pose, without compromising the general trajectory of the pose. For instance, in Paschimottanasana (Seated Forward Bend Pose), you might require more length in the lower back in order to prevent flexing (rounding) it. Bringing support closer or higher, whether it's a chair or bolster in front of you or sitting on support to raise the seat, reduces the reach in the pose.

The floor beneath you will prevent you from doing anything other than facing yourself, and so it goes with all BEING poses.

CHAPTER 3

BEING POSES: THE YAPANA WAY

I often hear from yoga students that practicing BEING poses have better prepared them for DOING, or classical poses. And yoga teachers often tell me they learn more about the DOING poses while working with students and their own bodies in the BEING poses. This happens because: The Whoever you are in any given DOING pose, however you avoid or overdue an area, presents itself quite loudly in the BEING poses. For instance, you can practice Utthita Trikonasana (Extended Triangle Pose) classically – standing upright in the middle of your mat. Any difficulties with front leg alignment, femur rotation, hamstring flexibility, or perhaps a neutral pelvis position, will show up in the BEING version of the pose. But this time, you will have to address the challenges. The floor beneath you will prevent you from doing anything other than facing yourself, and so it goes with all BEING poses.

The support that is required sheds light on what is or isn't happening when practicing the pose classically, and in a BEING variation, can skillfully guide the outcome of any change necessary. BEING poses require little or no effort, meaning that they do not recruit the same level of muscle effort as DOING poses, other than getting into the pose and maintaining limb alignment. They are generally considered cooling poses.

AWAKENING: BACKBENDS

A yoga backbend should have these three things: A stable structure, soft lines to its shape, and ample open space. In theory, it should also rival the suspension of the Brooklyn Bridge.

There are two classifications of yoga poses some may turn away from or fear. Consider a few commonly used phrases: "It was a real back bender" or "I bent over backwards for her." Each has negative connotations, but more importantly they convey that back bending is unpleasant. The truth is, back bending is unpleasant when done incorrectly, unsafely, and without an understanding of the biomechanics. Prone backbends are different than supine backbends. The great thing about practicing backbends restoratively is that they can be targeted to address your specific challenges without overloading any one segment of the spine. You can gain spinal flexibility without undue stress on the discs. Having said that, weight-bearing backbends are equally as important when practiced safely to promote strong and healthy bones.

A range of emotions may surface while practicing BEING backbends, but they are not to be forced. Rather, these supported poses can be an opportunity to evoke a deep acceptance in matters of the heart, or simply receiving the moment as it arises with whatever it may bring. BEING backbend poses encourage a slow and steady opening in the chest and front body. These supported relaxing backbends may appear as if not much is going on compared to DOING backbend poses, however, looks are deceiving. Backbends are the most energetic of the BEING poses. They stretch small spinal muscles groups over time, but because they do not recruit any effort at all they are also relaxing – just breathing, feeling and sensing.

General Contraindications

- Serious back, neck, shoulder, or knee injury – consult a qualified yoga therapist
- Insomnia
- Migraine
- Recent abdominal or chest surgery

General Benefits

- Keeps spine flexible
- Massages and stimulates organs
- Good for digestion
- Good release and re-patterning for hyper-kyphosis
- Good for depression – proceed slowly and with caution
- Good for asthma – proceed slowly and with caution

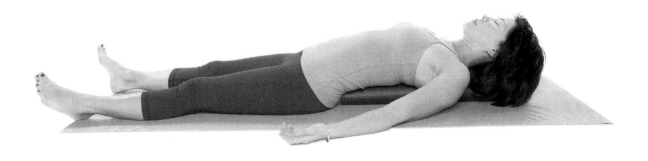

BASIC MATSYASANA (FISH POSE)

How to move into Basic Matsyasana

1. Roll a thin yoga mat from the short side.
2. Place the short end of the mat up against the spine, either at the lower back or behind the back ribs. Be sure to support the head.
3. Stretch out the legs and arms.
4. Breathe and relax.

How to come out of Basic Matsyasana

1. Release the arms if they are stretched overhead.
2. Bend the knees and set the feet onto the floor.
3. Draw the left arm into the chest.
4. Push off the feet and roll to the right side.
5. Pause.
6. Prepare for what's next.

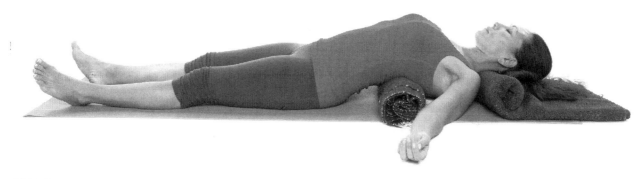

MATSYASANA, VAR. 1

How to move into Matsyasana, Var. 1

In this variation the blankets are rolled to support the level of opening you wish to receive in the chest and neck.

1. Position two long-rolled blankets behind you and across the mat, approximately 1 foot away from each other.
2. Sit with your knees bent in front of the first blanket and while using your hands for support, lie back until the shoulder blades rest across the blanket, the arms fit between the two blankets, and the neck or head is supported on the second blanket.
3. Stretch the legs out and keep them hip-width distance apart. Allow the arms to relax with the palms turned upward.
4. Relax the front bottom ribs.
5. Allow the arms to relax with the palms turned upward.
6. Breathe and relax.

How to come out of Matsyasana, Var. 1

1. Follow the Basic pose instructions.

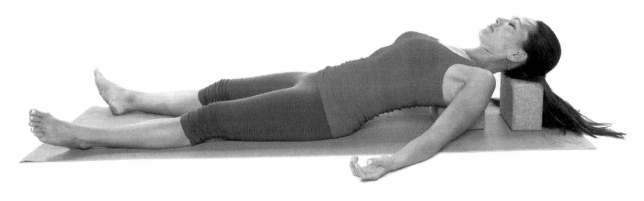

MATSYASANA, VAR. 2

How to move into Matsyasana, Var. 2

Two blocks are used in this variation to provide solid support for the mid and upper back. The blocks can be oriented on the flat wide side, or the thin side. The flat side of the block placed at the mid back provides superficial support against the muscles. While placing the block at the thin side offers more feedback against the spinal ligaments of the mid back. The highest orientation of the block provides the most amount of stimulation.

1. Position two yoga blocks at the top of the yoga mat; one on the wide, flat side and the other on the long thin side.
2. With your knees bent, sit in front of the block resting on its wide, flat side, and while using your hands for support, lie back until the shoulder blades rest across the block and the head rests on the other block.
3. Stretch the legs out and keep them hip-width distance apart.
4. Allow the arms to relax with the palms turned upward.
5. Relax the front bottom ribs.
6. Breathe and relax.

How to come out of Matsyasana, Var. 2

1. Follow the Basic pose instructions.

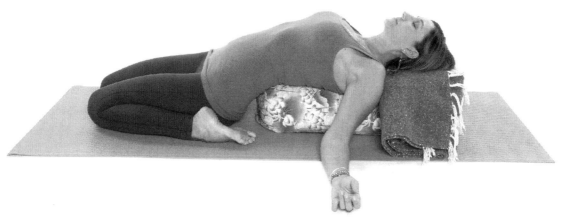

BASIC SUPTA VIRASANA (RECLINING HERO POSE)

This backbend gives a big stretch to the front thigh muscles (quadriceps), knees, and ankles. This pose is not for everyone, because it extends the lower back. This is a pose that can be worked up to once the quadriceps are flexible and you have had considerable experience with backbends. However, simply build up the support and increase the angle (Reduce the Reach) so that the pose comes to you rather than you trying to get to the pose. The short end of the bolster can be placed right up against the lower back or lower back ribs. Some people prefer the support at the lower back, while others feel compressed and require the lift at the ribs.

How to move into Basic Supta Virasana

1. Kneel in front of a bolster positioned parallel to and at the top end of the mat with a long-folded blanket on the top end of the bolster.
2. Use the hands to stretch the calf muscles away from the knees and toward the heels.
3. Drop the hips to sit on the floor with the hips between each foot.
4. Place the hands on the feet to use the arms as leverage to lift the chest and safely lie back on the bolster, resting the head on the blanket.
5. Lift and broaden the chest.
6. Breathe and relax.

How to come out of Basic Supta Virasana

1. Gently tuck the chin.
2. Push the hands into the feet or against the floor to use as leverage to lift up and out of the pose.
3. Pause.
4. Prepare for what's next.

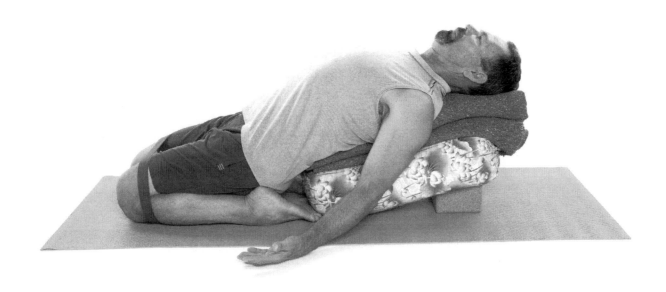

SUPTA VIRASANA, VAR. 1

Try this variation if you need a little more relief in the lower back. Notice how the top end of the bolster is elevated with a block and the bolster has two double-folded blankets on top to bring further height (Reduce the Reach) to the student.

How to move into Supta Virasana, Var. 1

1. Follow the Basic pose instructions with the modified prop placement.
2. Breathe and relax.

How to come out of Supta Virasana, Var. 1

1. Follow the Basic pose instructions.

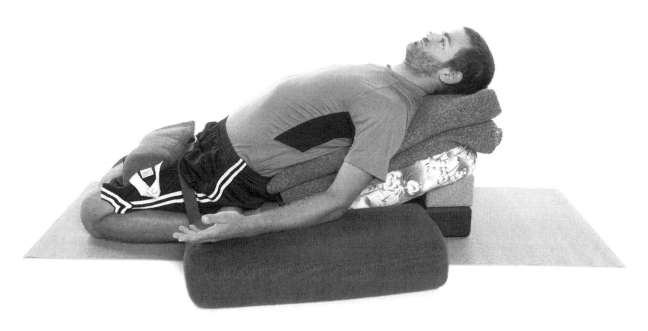

SUPTA VIRASANA, VAR 2

In this variation, the pose is considerably elevated in order to meet flexibility challenges. Doubled-folded blankets stacked as a bolster, with the short ends stair-stepped by approximately 1", rest on top of the bolster in order to better support the lower back.

How to move into Supta Virasana, Var. 2

1. Follow the Basic pose instructions with modified prop placement.
2. Breathe and relax.

How to come out of Supta Virasana, Var. 2

1. Follow the Basic pose instructions.

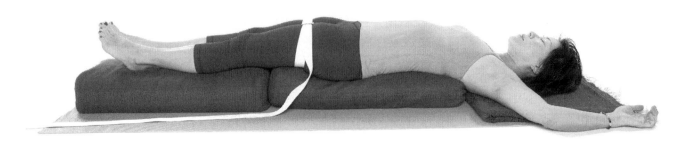

BASIC SETU BANDHA SARVANGASANA (RECLINING BRIDGE POSE)

This backbend keeps the heart above the head, so it is also considered a soft inversion that provides circulation of blood to the chest and neck. It lengthens the front center line of the body and is known for its therapeutic application for hypertension. A belt is fastened around the top thighs to keep them from separating while in the pose.

How to move into Basic Setu Bandha Sarvangasana

1. Prepare the set-up by lining up the short ends of two bolsters to make a "bed."
2. Sit on the bolsters with the knees bent and fasten a belt around the legs.
3. With the support of your hands and feet, slide back until your upper back, shoulders, and head are resting on the floor.
4. Place your arms into a goal post position, being sure to keep the backs of the shoulders flat on the ground.
5. Relax the front ribs.
6. Breathe and relax.

How to come out of Basic Setu Bandha Sarvangasana

1. Release the tension of the belt.
2. Bend the knees and place the feet on the ground alongside the bolster.
3. Push off the feet to slide the body back off and off of the support until the pelvis and lower back rest on the floor.
4. Draw the knees into the chest and roll to the side.
5. Pause.
6. Prepare for what's next.

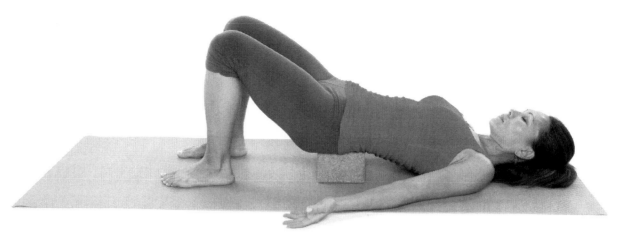

SETU BANDHA SARVANGASANA, VAR. 1

For more lift in the pelvis, the following three variations act as a stronger inversion with variations 2 and 3 offering the greatest elevation. The blocks help to stabilize the lower back and sacrum making them a good choice for those challenged with SI Joint Dysfunction, if stabilization is needed. The SI Joint is the connection between the spine and the pelvis. Too much or not enough movement in the joint results in inflammation. It supports the spine by providing stability and acts as a shock absorber for forces to the lower extremities.

How to move into Setu Bandha Sarvangasana, Var. 1

1. Lie back with a the knees bent.
2. Lift the hips and place a block on the flat wide side against the tailbone and sacrum.
3. Relax the arms alongside the body with the hands positioned approximately 6" away from the hips and the palms turned up.
4. Relax the shoulders and head.
5. Relax the front ribs.
6. Breathe and relax.

How to come out of Setu Bandha Sarvangasana, Var. 1

1. Lift hips away from the block and return the body to the ground, keeping the knees bent.
2. Pause.
3. Prepare for what's next.

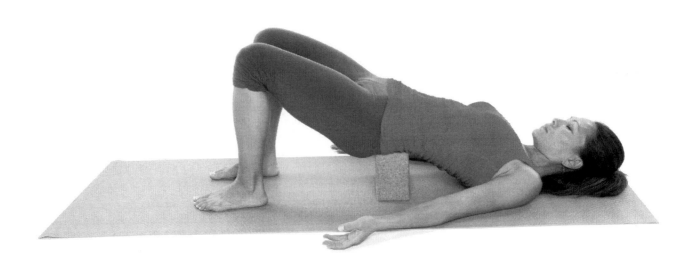

SETU BANDHA SARVANGASANA, VAR. 2

How to move into Setu Bandha Sarvangasana, Var. 2

1. Follow the Basic pose instructions with modified prop placement.
2. Breathe and relax.

How to come out of Setu Bandha Sarvangasana, Var. 2

1. Follow the pose instructions for variation 1.

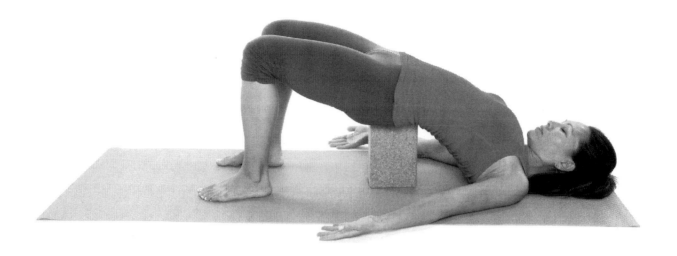

SETU BANDHA SARVANGASANA, VAR. 3

You can play with the height. You might even decide to explore more height than the photo below by placing a block on it's flat, wide side and stack another block on top of its long, thin side. Explore as you wish, but remember to keep both of the shoulders on the floor no matter how much your pelvis is elevated.

How to move into Setu Bandha Sarvangasana Var. 3

1. Follow the Basic pose instruction with modified prop placement.
2. Breathe and relax.

How to come out of Setu Bandha Sarvangasana, Var. 3

1. Follow the pose instructions for variation 2.

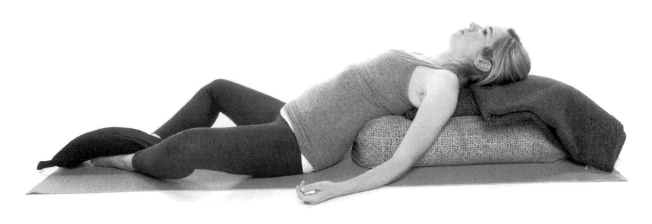

BASIC SUPTA BADDHA KONASANA (RECLINING BOUND ANGLE POSE)

A wonderful pose for the legs and hips. Be sure to support the upper legs if they are above hip level. This way there will not be an uneven load on the hips. The support provides good feedback for the legs to relax. Just like Supta Virasana (Reclining Hero Pose), the support at the back may be placed directly against the lower back, or at the back ribs. This is a pose that everyone can practice and I haven't met anyone who hasn't enjoyed being in it. Like all of the poses, it only needs to meet you where you are.

How to move into Basic Supta Baddha Konasana

1. Position a bolster parallel on your mat and one or two folded blankets at the top end of the bolster.
2. Sit in front of the short end of the bolster and bring the soles of the feet together so the knees fall to the sides.
3. Using your hands for support, gently lie back onto the support.
4. For additional "grounding" place a 10 lb. sandbag on the feet.
5. Allow the lower body to relax and sink into the floor and the upper body to open.
6. Breathe and relax.

How to come out of Basic Supta Baddha Konasana

1. Gently tuck the chin.
2. Use the hands as leverage against the floor to lift up and out of the pose.
3. Slide one foot out to the side and then straighten the leg, follow by the other leg.
4. Pause with the legs straight and sit upright.
5. Prepare for what's next.

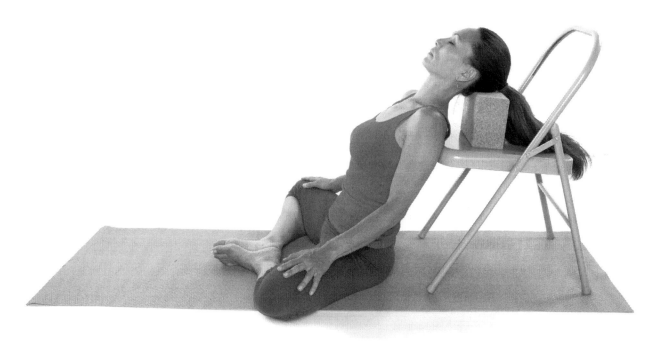

SUPTA BADDHA KONASANA, VAR. 1

This is a lovely way to get the opening in the mid back and legs without having to be in fully reclined position.

How to move into Supta Baddha Konasana, Var. 1

1. Position a chair on the yoga mat with a yoga block on the seat.
2. Sit in front of the chair and bring the soles of the feet together so the knees fall to the sides.
3. Using the hands for support, lift the chest while leaning back to rest the bottom of the shoulder blades against the front lip of the chair.
4. Rest your hands on the legs and your head on the block.
5. Sink the lower body into the floor and relax the front ribs.
6. Breathe and relax.

How to come out of Supta Baddha Konasana, Var. 1

1. Follow the Basic pose instructions.

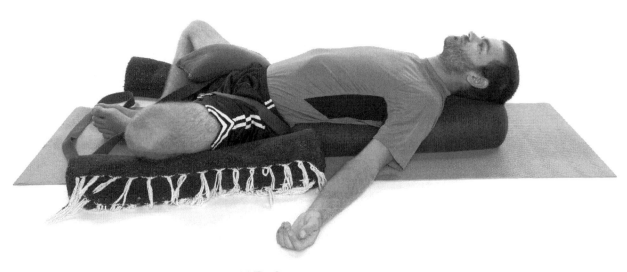

SUPTA BADDHA KONASANA, VAR. 2

Imbalances happen in all of us. One shoulder or hip is tighter than the other, or one segment of the spine is much weaker than the others. This variation shows how using a 10 lb. sandbag on the tighter leg can help to even out flexibility challenges. A yoga belt is fastened around the lower back and around the inner legs and outer feet in order to help stabilize the pelvis as it stretches out the lower body. And this variation shows the short end of the bolster positioned right against the lower back and without any blanket support on top of it. Long-rolled blankets are placed underneath the upper thighs and shins to support the stretch the legs of the stretch.

How to move into Supta Baddha Konasana, Var. 2

1. Follow the Basic pose instructions with modified prop placement.
2. Breathe and relax.

How to come out of Supta Baddha Konasana, Var. 2

1. Follow the Basic pose instructions.

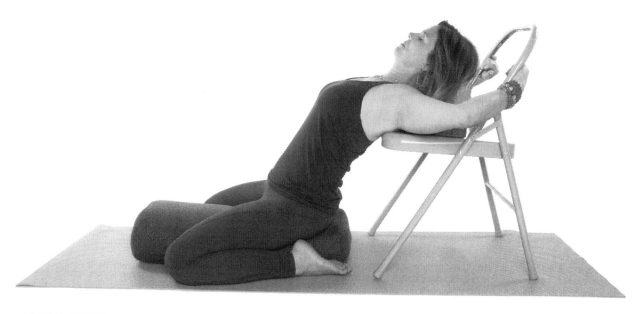

BASIC USTRASANA (CAMEL POSE)

This backbend is a good alternative for opening the chest in a seated position with a similar legs stretch done in classic Camel Pose, standing on the knees. Of course, you can change the leg position to your preference. This is a combination of Basic Virasana (Basic Hero Pose) in the lower body and Supta Baddha Konasana (Reclining Bound Angle Pose Variation 1) in the upper body. You can change the upper body and lower body positions to meet any criteria or creative urge.

How to move into Basic Ustrasana

1. Position a sturdy chair on the mat with a block on the seat, and a bolster half-way underneath the chair.
2. Straddle the bolster with your legs folded behind you and your back facing the chair.
3. Using the hands for support, lift the chest while leaning back to rest the bottom of the shoulder blades against the front lip of the chair.
4. Rest your hands on your thighs or hold onto the chair back rest for a deeper chest and shoulder stretch.
5. Relax the front ribs.
6. Breathe and relax.

How to come out of Basic Ustrasana

1. Gently tuck the chin.
2. Use the hands as leverage against the floor to lift up and out of the pose.
3. Breathe and relax.
3. Slide one foot out to the side and then straighten the leg, follow by the other leg.
4. Pause with the legs straight and sit upright.
5. Prepare for what's next.

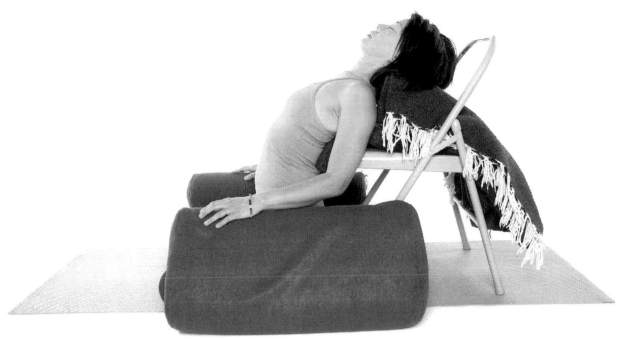

USTRASANA, VAR. 1

This variation offers additional lift in the mid back for those who may require it. If the you don't feel the chest "popping" in Basic Ustrasana or variation 1 (without the front ribs being aggressively pushed forward) this modification will provide it. Simply place a long-folded blanket and drape over the front lip of the chair and block which the head will rest on. Positioning two bolsters on either side of the hips creates the perfect hand rest.

How to move into Ustrasana, Var. 1

1. Follow the Basic pose instructions with modified prop placement.

How to come out of Ustrasana, Var. 1

1. Follow the Basic pose instructions.

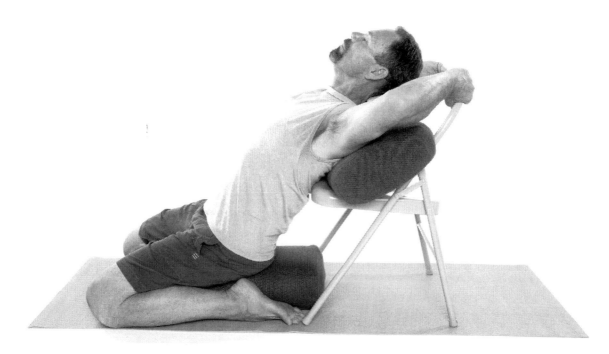

USTRASANA, VAR. 2

For less of a mid and upper backbend, a bolster is placed on top of the chair to meet flexibility challenges (Reduce the Reach). The angle of the bolster supports the back of the shoulder and the shoulder blades. This allows tight shoulders to stretch without compromising safe alignment.

How to move into Ustrasana, Var. 2

1.   Follow the Basic pose instructions with modified prop placement.

How to come out of Ustrasana, Var. 2

1.   Follow the Basic pose instructions.

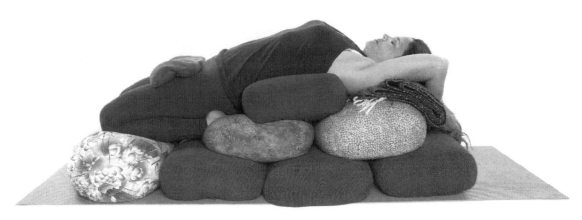

BASIC BACK VIPARITA DANDASANA (INVERTED TWO LEGGED STAFF POSE)

If you have a lot of bolsters, this backbend provides ample support to all segments of the spine. Be sure to follow the instructions for coming out. Curling up out of the pose or rolling to one side puts to much load on the back. Instead, you'll slide your way out head first and enjoy every minute of it.

How to move into Basic Viparita Dandasana

1. Position three bolsters next to each other across the mat.
2. Stack two more bolsters, centered, on top.
3. Stack one more bolster on top, centered, so the shape looks similar to a pyramid.
4. Position a meditation pad or double-folded blanket just behind the head-side of the bolster.
5. Fasten a belt around the top thighs.
6. Using your hands for support, sit on the bolster of the second row.
7. Lean back so the lower and mid back are supported by the top center bolster and the neck waterfalls off the back edge of the top bolster.
8. Stretch the arms overhead shoulder distance apart with the palms facing each other.
9. Bend the elbows and tuck the palms behind the bolster beneath you and keep the elbows shoulder distance apart.
10. Breathe and relax.

How to come out of Basic Viparita Dandasana

1. Release the arms from overhead.
2. Place your hands against the bottom bolsters.
3. Bend your knees and place the feet onto the floor.
4. Tuck your chin and push your hands and feet to slowly and with control, roll off the support in the direction of your head until your lower back and hips touch the floor and your lower legs rest on the support.
5. Pause.
6. Prepare for what's next.

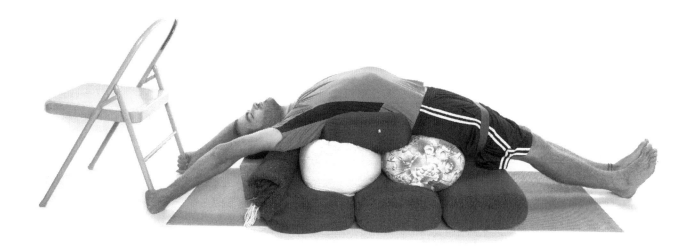

VIPARITA DANDASANA, VAR. 1

In this variation, the shoulders are in full flexion behind the head, but holding onto the legs of the chair supports the shoulders for safe alignment while stretching them. A block has replaced a blanket for the head to rest on to adapt to body length. This is similar to being stretched on a rack – in a good way! It offers tremendous traction to unfurl any tight spots in the back.

How to move into Viparita Dandasana, Var. 1

1. Follow the Basic pose instructions with modified prop placement.
2. Breathe and relax.

How to come out of Viparita Dandasana, Var. 1

1. Follow the Basic pose instructions.

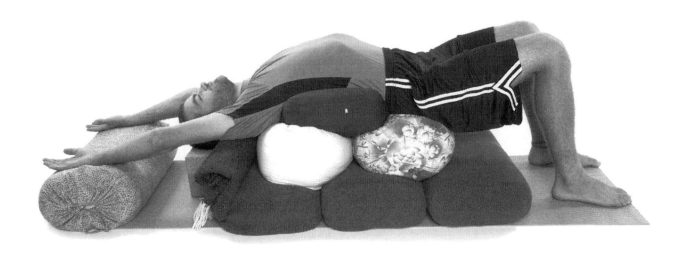

VIPARITA DANDASANA, VAR. 2

If the extension on the lower back is too much simply bend the knees and place the feet flat on the floor. If the flexion of the arms are too much, the head will drop below the shoulders and the shoulder joints may impinge. In this case, it's best to support the head with a block to keep it in the same plane as the shoulders and position a bolster underneath the forearms and hands.

How to move into Viparita Dandasana, Var. 2

1. Follow the Basic pose instructions with modified prop placement.
2. Breathe and relax.

How to come out of Viparita Dandasana, Var. 2

1. Follow the Basic pose instructions.

*Yapana BEING twists are calming to the nervous system
and improve vertebral joint flexibility.*

CHAPTER 4
UNWINDING: TWISTS

BEING twist poses involve opposing movements; a straight line is maintained in the spine while the pelvis and shoulder girdles stack. They can be practiced as a wringing out movement, where more emphasis is placed on rotation, or a spiral movement with more emphasis on thoracic extension. In either case, torque on the lumbar should be avoided and more focus on thoracic rotation should be given. You can begin your practice with a twist as long as it is followed by a pose that puts the spine in a neutral position, such as Child Pose, Half Knee to Chest Pose, or a forward bend – anything that doesn't rotate or bend it right away.

Miraculously, BEING twists seem to untether the knots stored in the back. Many students, after practicing BEING twists, experience the unwinding of accumulated stress. BEING twists are calming to the nervous system and improve vertebral joint flexibility.

General Contraindications

- Sciatica
- Sacroiliac Joint Dysfunction
- Herniated discs
- Pregnancy
- Recent abdominal surgery

General Benefits

- Improve vertebral joint flexibility
- Good for digestion
- Squeeze and soak the internal organs

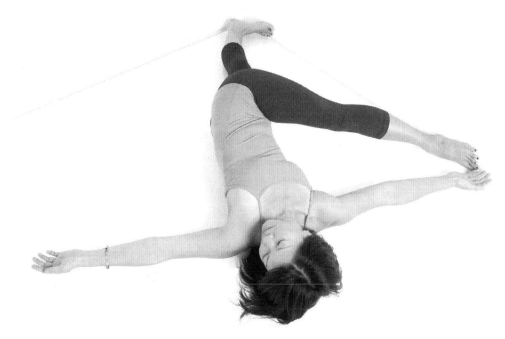

BASIC SUPTA PARIVRTTA TRIKONASANA
(BASIC RECLINING REVOLVED TRIANGLE POSE)

This is a supine (on the back) take on the classic standing version: Revolved Triangle Pose. This deep twist can be practiced with a "wringing out" or "spiral" movement in the thoracic. Play with the two to see which offers you the most opening without disturbing the lower back. The bag should be placed across the front of the shoulder and upper arm and not placed on a shoulder that is elevated more than 1" away from the floor. Both shoulders must remain on floor and the hips stacked, so it's not important to reach the bottom hand to the foot. Just move in that direction.

How to move into Basic Supta Parivrtta Trikonasana

1. Lie on the right side of the body in a 90° position like Chair Pose,
    with the feet stacked near a wall.
2. Reach the left leg forward and the right leg behind you into a "scissor" legged shape.
3. Slide the body to the right, reaching the right hand toward the left foot.
4. Straighten the legs while turning the torso open so the back rests flat on the floor.
5. Make small adjustments to find the classic shape of the pose against the floor.
6. Breathe and relax.

How to come out of Basic Supta Parivrtta Trikonasana

1. Draw both the back leg and arm into the body's center and roll to the right.
2. Pause.
3. Prepare for the opposite side.

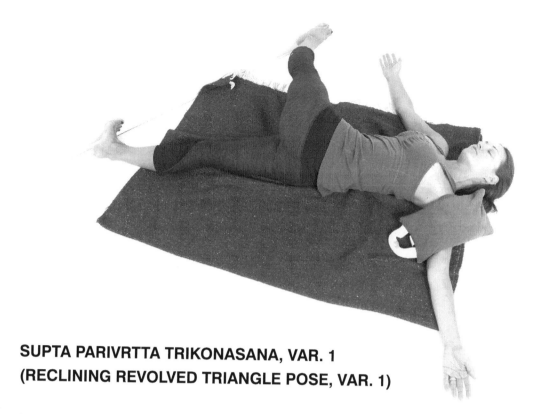

SUPTA PARIVRTTA TRIKONASANA, VAR. 1
(RECLINING REVOLVED TRIANGLE POSE, VAR. 1)

How to move into Supta Parivrtta Trikonasana, Var. 1

1. Follow the Basic pose instructions with modified prop placement.
2. Breathe and relax.

Using a 10 lb. sandbag keeps the top shoulder "grounded" and provides that extra bit of opening to a tight chest. Only consider using this prop when the shoulder is already touching the floor. The bag should be placed across the front of the shoulder and upper arm. Avoid placing the bag on the neck or elbow. And remember to keep the hips stacked so the top hip is not rolling forward of the bottom one. This ensures a steady pelvis for encouraging the twist in the mid back rather than the lower back.

How to come out of Supta Parivrtta Trikonasana, Var. 1

1. Follow the Basic pose instructions.

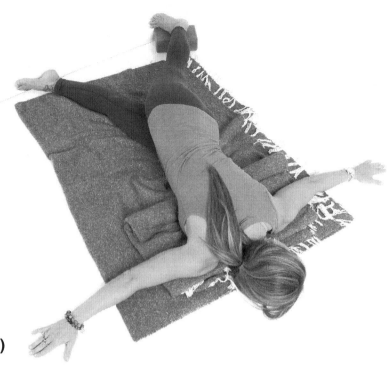

SUPTA PARIVRTTA TRIKONASANA, VAR. 2

(RECLINING REVOLVED TRIANGLE POSE, VAR. 2)

If your mid-back is fairly loose, you might try this variation. A block can be placed at the wall and underneath the back foot to promote hip separation, which helps to better stack the hips and prevent the top leg from collapsing. In this photo below, I've placed half of a long-rolled blanket underneath the chest. This additional support may be desirable for some women.

How to move into Supta Parivrtta Trikonasana, Var. 2

1. Lie on the right side of the body with slightly bent knees with the feet stacked near a wall.
2. Step the right foot forward and the left foot behind you into a short "scissor" legged shape.
3. Press the hands on the floor and push away from it to lift and turn the torso to the right.
4. Stretch the arms out into a "T" position so they are perpendicular to the torso and turn the head to the right.
5. Make small adjustments to find the classic shape of the pose against the floor.
6. Breathe and relax.

How to come out of Supta Parivrtta Trikonasana, Var. 2

1. Turn the head to the left.
2. Bend both knees and draw them into your center.
3. Pause.
4. Prepare for the opposite side.

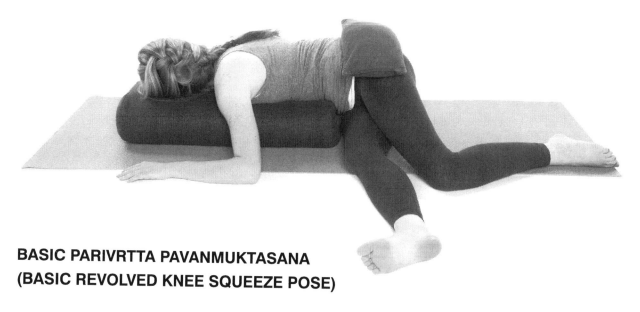

BASIC PARIVRTTA PAVANMUKTASANA (BASIC REVOLVED KNEE SQUEEZE POSE)

This relaxing twist targets the turn of the belly. Because it is a prone (on the belly) twist, the height of the support should allow for the hips and shoulders to be in the same plane. Also, keep the elbows and shoulders in the same plane. First, draw the shoulders down and away from the ears so they aren't hiking up to the neck. Keeping the arms in a 90° position will prevent the shoulders and shoulder blades from lifting.

How to move into Basic Parivrtta Pavanmuktasana

1. Position a bolster parallel on the mat.
2. Sit the right hip against the short end of the bolster and bend the left leg behind you.
3. Place your hands on either side of the bolster, push them into the floor using it as leverage to lift the chest and rotate it and the head to the right side.
4. Lower the torso onto the bolster.
5. Place the arms in a "goal post" position.
6. Breathe and relax.
7. Lower the torso onto the bolster.

How to come out of Basic Parivrtta Pavanmuktasana

1. Keep the chin in a neutral position relative to a neutral skull and turn the head to rest the forehead on the bolster.
2. Place the hands on the floor underneath the shoulders.
3. Push the hands into the floor to straighten the arms and lift the torso away from the bolster.
4. Straighten both legs and sit upright.
5. Pause.
6. Prepare for the opposite side.

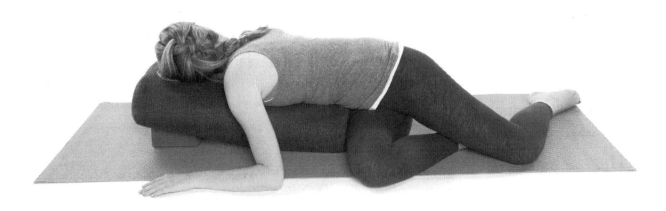

PARIVRTTA PAVANMUKTASANA, VAR. 1
(REVOLVED KNEE SQUEEZE POSE, VAR. 1)

A simple way to keep the shoulders and hips in the same plane is to elevate the top end of the bolster as in this variation. Unlike the Basic version, the top leg here is bent, which decreases the stretch of the leg and the lower back.

How to move into Parivrtta Pavanmuktasana, Var. 1

1. Follow the Basic pose instructions with modified prop placement.
2. Breathe and relax.

How to come out of Parivrtta Pavanmuktasana, Var. 1

1. Follow the Basic pose instructions.

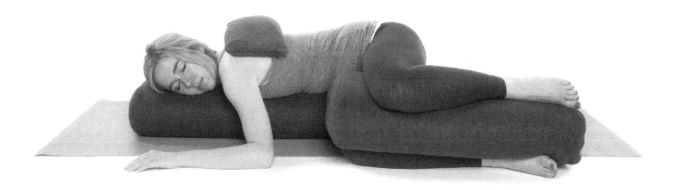

PARIVRTTA PAVANMUKTASANA, VAR. 2
(REVOLVED KNEE SQUEEZE POSE, VAR. 2)

In some cases, tight or short neck and upper back muscles prevent us from easily turning the head away from the knees. Simply turning the head in the direction of the knees resolves this and placing a 10 lb. sandbag across the shoulder blades. Just that little bit of weight can help relax the muscles so the shoulders stay in the same plane. This allows the weight of the twist to remain even rather than loading on one side of the body.

How to move into Parivrtta Pavanmuktasana, Var. 2

1.   Follow the basic pose instructions with modified prop placement.
2.   Breathe and relax.

How to come out of Parivrtta Pavanmuktasana, Var. 2

1.   Follow the Basic pose instructions.

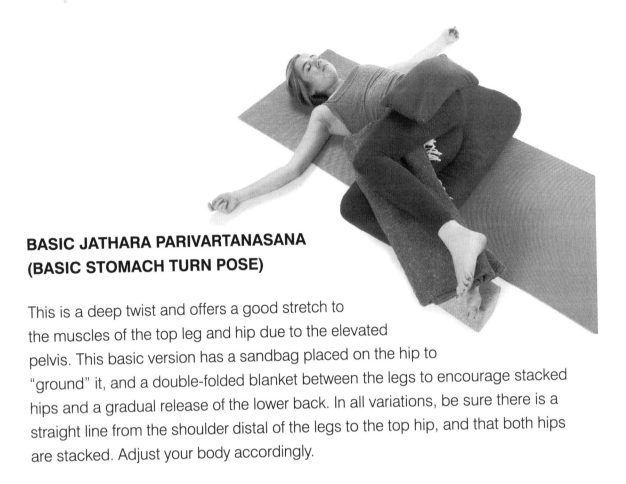

BASIC JATHARA PARIVARTANASANA (BASIC STOMACH TURN POSE)

This is a deep twist and offers a good stretch to the muscles of the top leg and hip due to the elevated pelvis. This basic version has a sandbag placed on the hip to "ground" it, and a double-folded blanket between the legs to encourage stacked hips and a gradual release of the lower back. In all variations, be sure there is a straight line from the shoulder distal of the legs to the top hip, and that both hips are stacked. Adjust your body accordingly.

How to move into Basic Jathara Parivartanasana

1. Position a bolster across the mat, a block approximately 1' in front of the bolster, and have folded blankets and a block nearby.
2. Lie down on your back with the arms in a "T" position and lift the hips to rest your lower back and pelvis on the bolster.
3. Push your feet into the floor, lift the hips again and scoot them to the far left of the bolster.
4. Place a double-folded blanket between the legs and as you lower the knees to the right, rest the feet on the block.
5. Place a sandbag on the top hip.
6. Breathe and relax.

How to come out of Basic Jathara Parivartanasana

1. Draw the top knee into the chest, keeping it close to the torso as you move.
2. Draw the opposite knee into the chest.
3. When both knees are in toward the chest, place the feet on the floor.
4. Rest the pelvis and lower back on the center of the bolster.
5. Pause.
6. Prepare for the opposite side.

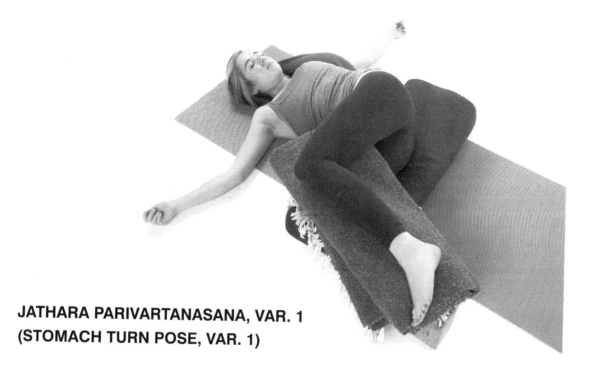

JATHARA PARIVARTANASANA, VAR. 1
(STOMACH TURN POSE, VAR. 1)

Remember, all twists require both shoulders to be resting on the floor to promote a well-balanced rotation in the spine and prevent overloading on one side of the body. If your back muscles are tight the shoulder farthest from the knees will likely lift away from the floor. The sandbag supports the shoulder to "ground" and gently coaches the back muscles and shoulder to relax into gravity. A sandbag should not be placed on a shoulder that is elevated more than 1" away from the floor.

How to move into Jathara Parivartanasana, Var. 1

1. Follow the Basic pose instructions with modified prop placement.
2. Breathe and relax.

How to come out of Jathara Parivartanasana, Var. 1

1. Follow the Basic pose instructions.

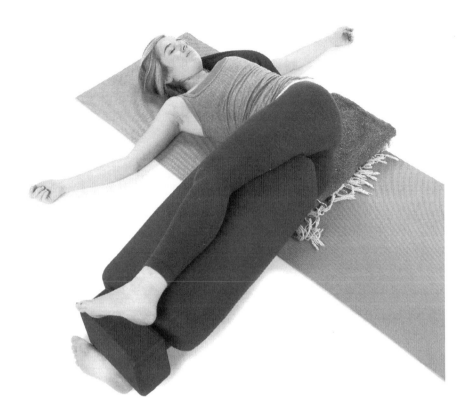

JATHARA PARIVARTANASANA, VAR. 2
(STOMACH TURN POSE, VAR. 2)

This variation offers the strongest of sensations by straightening both legs. Straightening both legs offers additional stretch to the lower back and legs. A bolster and block has been placed between the legs to keep the hips stacked, and a sandbag on the shoulder to keep them in the same plane. The bottom support has been replaced with a double-folded blanket. Breathe into this one!

How to move into Jathara Parivartanasana, Var. 2

1. Follow the Basic pose instructions with modified prop placement.
2. Breathe and relax.

How to come out of Jathara Parivartanasana, Var. 2

1. Follow the Basic pose instructions.

Yapana supported inversion poses are the easiest way
to invert the body with the least amount of work.

CHAPTER 5
DECOMPRESSING: INVERSIONS

Yapana BEING Inversion poses are the easiest way to invert the body with the least amount of work. They are excellent variations with the same benefits as DOING inversions, and can be practiced by anyone that is a candidate for inverting.

Going upside down can be scary for some people even when the pose is well supported. Consider trying the inverted BEING poses that are the least threatening, like "Legs Up the Chair", then graduate toward stronger inversions.

General Contraindications

- Vertigo
- Headache
- Serious heart problems
- Heavy menstruation –
  first days of heavy bleeding
- Uncontrolled high blood pressure
  and heart conditions
- Detached retina
- Inflammation of eyes and ears
- Pulled hamstrings – proceed with caution
- Pregnancy – after the first trimester and only
  if the student has a regular inversion practice
  and is comfortable with inverting. Pregnant
  women are known to become very in-tune with
  their body. Follow your instincts.

General Benefits

- Helps to reverse the effects of gravity
- Relieves tired legs and feet
- Encourages venous return
  (keeps fluids moving toward the heart)
- Refreshes the brain with freshly
  oxygenated blood
- Calms the mind

BASIC VIPARITA KARANI
(BASIC "LEGS UP THE WALL" POSE)

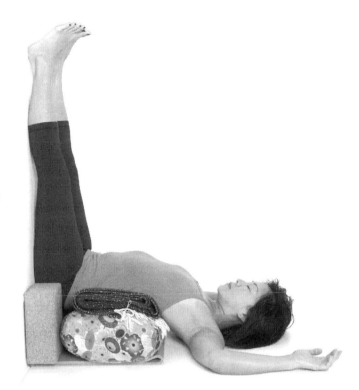

Here's an inverted pose that I always practice when traveling. After I settle into my hotel room, I slide my legs up the wall. Many times, I've fallen asleep while in this pose. You don't need a lot of props for this one – really, just a wall will do. The shoulders should remain on the floor with the legs straight. For a bigger backbend, place a folded blanket on top of the bolster. Of course, you can modify the height of the pelvis from no support at all to a bolster and several blankets. You decide what makes sense and supports a smooth and steady breath.

How to move into Basic Viparita Karani

1. Fold a mat into thirds and place the long side against the wall.
2. Position two blocks with the flat, wide side against the wall, lined up with the outer edges of the mat.
3. Lie down on the floor with the pelvis between the two blocks and the legs up the wall.
4. Bend the knees, push the feet against the wall to lift the pelvis, and slide a bolster underneath the pelvis and lower back.
5. Bring your arms into a goal post or "T" position.
6. Breathe and relax.

How to come out of Basic Viparita Karani

1. Bend the knees, pushing the feet against the wall, and slide backwards until the pelvis and lower back are resting on the bolster.
2. Pause.
3. Slide back again until the pelvis and lower back are resting on the floor.
4. Pause.
5. Prepare for what's next.

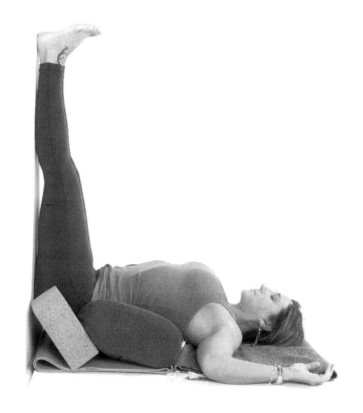

VIPARITA KARANI ("LEGS UP THE WALL" POSE, VAR. 1)

If your lower back is more flat than arched, this variation is a simple modification that supports the spine in the architecture of this particular pose. The angled blocks and bolster create a slight arch in the lower back. A blanket underneath the shoulders and head may be necessary to fill any daylight there might be between the two. Keep thinking how you can bring the pose to the student, not the student to the pose.

How to move into Viparita Karani, Var. 1

1. Follow the Basic pose instructions with modified prop placement.
2. Breathe and relax.

How to come out of Viparita Karani, Var. 1

1. Bend the knees and place the feet against the wall.
2. Push off the feet to lift the hips off the bolster.
3. Release the pelvis and lower back onto the floor.
4. Draw the knees into the chest and roll to one side.
5. Pause.
6. Prepare for what's next.

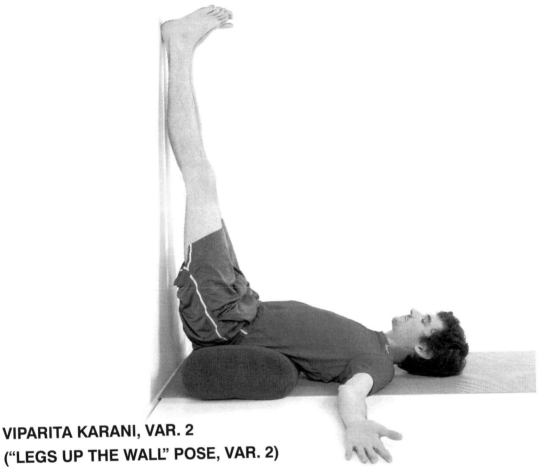

VIPARITA KARANI, VAR. 2
("LEGS UP THE WALL" POSE, VAR. 2)

Tight hamstrings (upper back leg muscles) will prevent you from bringing the legs flush to the wall. In the variation, the pelvis and legs do not rest directly against the wall (Reduce the Reach). If you attempt this pose with tight hamstrings and a posterior tilted pelvis, you will likely not be able to hold yourself on the support without effort. More importantly, the lower back is likely to flex, which should be avoided here.

How to move into Viparita Karani, Var. 2

1. Lie down on the floor and bring the pelvis either against a wall or about 5" to 6" away, resting the legs up the wall.
2. Bend the knees, push the feet against the wall to lift the pelvis and slide a bolster underneath the pelvis and lower back.
3. Bring your arms into a "T" position with the palms turned up.
4. Release the weight of your legs into the pelvis, and the pelvis into the bolster.
5. Breathe and relax.

How to come out of Viparita Karani, Var. 2

1. Follow the Viparita Karani, Var. 1 instructions.

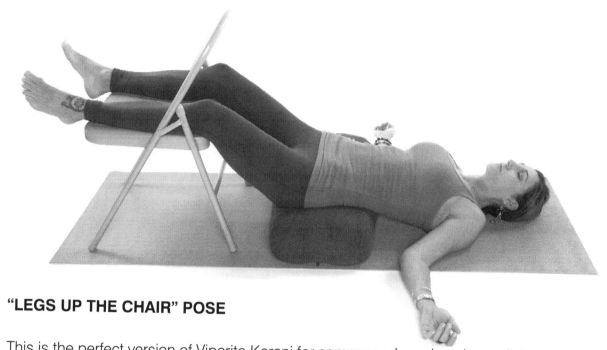

"LEGS UP THE CHAIR" POSE

This is the perfect version of Viparita Karani for someone whose legs keep sliding down the wall due to either very loose ligaments or very tight hamstrings. It can be practiced using similar modifications as we did in Viparita Karani, with a bolster, a bolster and folded blanket, or without any of it. And it's a nice option for someone who prefers less of an inversion.

BASIC "LEGS UP THE CHAIR" POSE

This is the mini variation of Viparita Karani ("Legs Up The Wall Pose). The only difference is that the lower legs are resting on a chair rather than stretched straight up a wall.

How to move into Basic "Legs Up The Chair" Pose

1. Position a sturdy chair on the mat with the seat of the chair facing you.
2. Have a bolster nearby.
3. Lie on your back and rest the lower legs on the seat of the chair with the backs of the knees touching the lip of the seat.
4. Press the lower legs into the seat of the chair to lift the hips up, then slide the bolster underneath the pelvis and lower back.
5. Allow the lower body to sink into gravity.
6. Breathe and relax.

How to come out of Basic "Legs Up The Chair" Pose

1. Lift the hips to remove any support underneath them.
2. Draw the knees into the chest.
3. Roll to one side.
4. Pause.
5. Prepare for what's next.

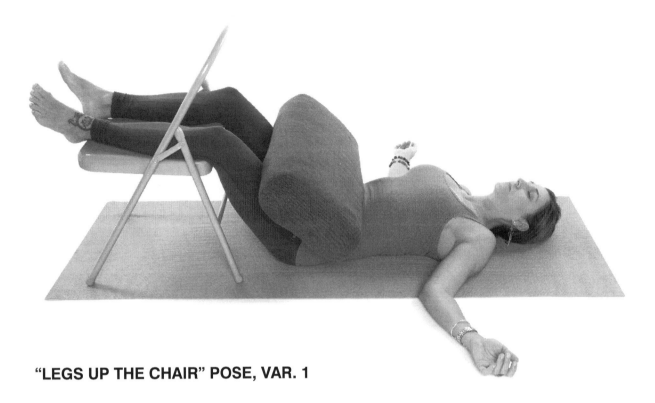

"LEGS UP THE CHAIR" POSE, VAR. 1

A little bit of weight on the top thighs helps to "ground" the lower back. This is a nice option for someone who has an achy lower back. The added weight helps to relax the lower back muscles. This is typically a valid option for everyone.

How to move into "Legs Up The Chair" Pose, Var. 1

1. Follow the Basic pose instructions with modified prop placement.
2. Breathe and relax.

How to come out of "Legs Up The Chair" Pose, Var. 1

1. Follow the Basic pose instructions.

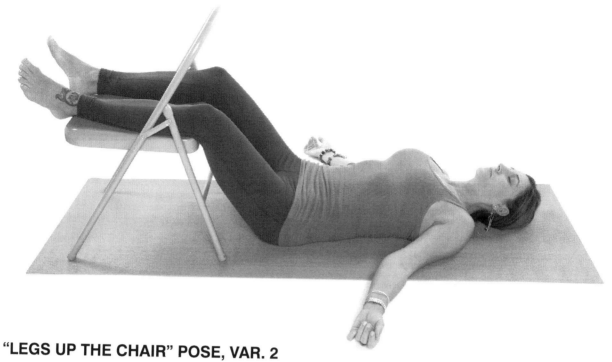

"LEGS UP THE CHAIR" POSE, VAR. 2

This is a simple way to relieve lower body fatigue and melt away the daily stressors.

How to move into "Legs Up The Chair" Pose, Var. 2

1. Follow the Basic pose instructions with modified prop placement.
2. Breathe and relax.

How to come out of "Legs Up The Chair" Pose, Var. 2

1. Follow the Basic pose instructions.

*Yapana forward bends are designed to cool the central nervous system
and to deeply promote the "rest and digest" response.*

CHAPTER 6
CALMING: FORWARD BENDS

The Yapana BEING forward bend poses can create space in the hips, pelvis, and lower back. They may be very challenging for beginning students with a posterior tilted pelvis, tight hamstrings, hip flexors, or lower back. Because they are designed to cool the central nervous system and to deeply promote "rest and digest," strategic prop placement is crucial for maintaining SAS and physical comfort in the pose. Sometimes you may have to make the choice of giving up something to get something else. Ask yourself: What is the purpose the forward bend serves? Your answer will determine the direction you pursue.

Three important rules are to be followed when practicing forward bends:

1. **Extension** – The pose must have two-thirds extension of the spine going into the pose before allowing flexion. For instance, the lower back must lengthen, not flex and round, two-thirds into the pose. After that, the mid back can flex as much as needed, however, it is recommended that the chest and sternum move forward to lengthen the back body as much as comfortable.

2. **Armless** – Keep the arms out of the equation. Do not use them to reach forward beyond the initial entry into the pose. There is no "achieving" in a BEING pose. Instead, use the props to support the arms if necessary so that they are not hovering above ground or holding onto the feet to increase the stretch.

3. **Lower Legs** – The lower legs do not need to be firm to maintain alignment and SAS, but they should be held straight on their centerlines to prevent collapsing out to the sides. The head should ALWAYS be supported in forward bends. This is an important component to the level of relaxation in all BEING forward bends. Releasing the weight of the head into gravity in a downward position prevents the neck and upper back muscles from firing to hold up its weight in the forward bend position. This is calming to the front of the brain.

General Contraindications

- Hamstring injury – consult a qualified yoga therapist
- Sciatica – proceed with caution
- Sacroiliac joint dysfunction
- Pregnancy – avoid constricting the abdomen

General Benefits

- Calms the brain
- Improves digestion
- Reduces fatigue
- Good for high blood pressure

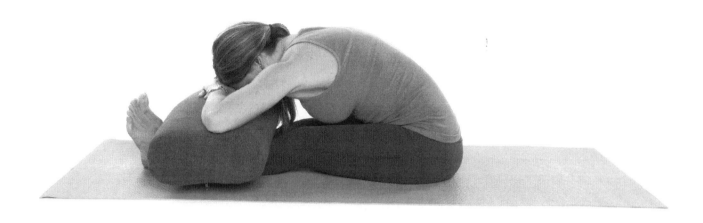

BASIC PASCHIMOTTANASANA
(BASIC SEATED FORWARD BEND POSE)

If your Hip Hinge is healthy you don't need a lot of support to be comfortable and still.

How to move into Basic Paschimottanasana

1. Sit upright and directly on the buttock bones with a bolster across the lower legs.
2. Lift the arms up alongside the head while keeping the lower ribs in and down.
3. Hinge forward at the hips while keeping your weight of the lower body sinking into the floor.
4. Hold onto the legs or feet while initially working the spine forward and down, keeping a flat back two-thirds of the way down before flexing.
5. Stretch both sides of the trunk evenly forward and relax the forehead on the arms or the bolster.
6. Breathe and relax.

How to come out of Basic Paschimottanasana

1. Lift out of the pose either with a flat back or rolling out vertebrae by vertebrae.
2. Pause.
3. Prepare for what's next.

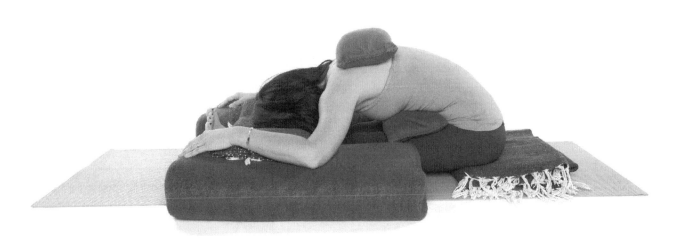

PASCHIMOTTANASANA VAR. 1
(SEATED FORWARD BEND POSE, VAR. 1)

The strongest of the variations, this option is great for someone with excellent flexibility who wishes to drop deep into the fold. There are two sandbags; one placed across the shoulder blades for added release to the upper back and shoulders, and one placed at the top thighs to weight down the legs and pelvis. To make sure the head is in the same plane as the chest, a doubled-folded blanket has been placed underneath the head. Bolsters are placed on either side of the legs and are used as arm support. If you have the flexibility and stability for this variation, two words: GO INSIDE.

How to move into Paschimottanasana, Var. 1

1. Follow the Basic pose instructions with modified prop placement.
2. Breathe and relax.

How to come out of Paschimottanasana, Var. 1

1. Follow the Basic pose instructions.

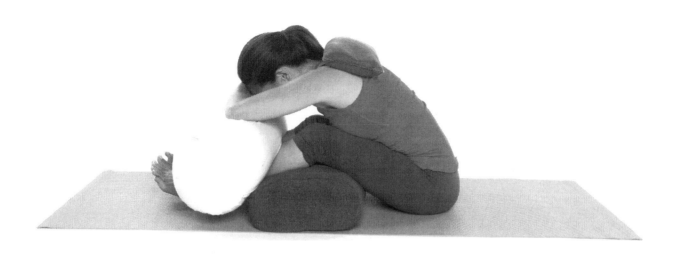

PASCHIMOTTANASANA VAR. 2
(SEATED FORWARD BEND POSE, VAR. 2)

Using the bolster underneath the knees and thighs supports tight hamstrings and offers a mild mid-back stretch. This variation, however, only makes sense if you can sit forward on the buttock bones. This really is the key to moving from the hips (Hip Hinge) rather than the lower back. You must be able to sit upright with your weight toward the front of the buttock bones, indicating that the pelvis is either in a neutral or anterior starting position. Another bolster is placed on top of the lower legs so the arms and head can rest rather than reach.

How to move into Paschimottanasana, Var. 2

1. Follow the Basic pose instructions with modified prop placement.
2. Breathe and relax.

How to come out of Paschimottanasna, Var. 2

1. Follow the Basic pose instructions.

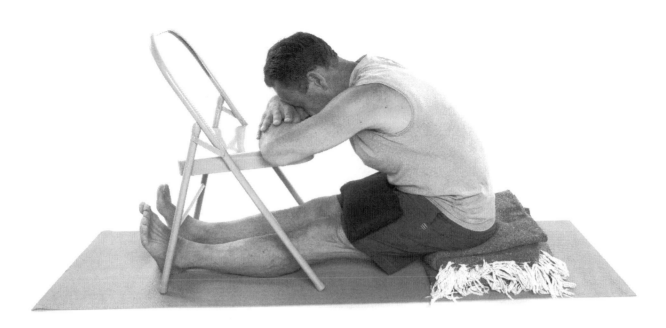

PASCHIMOTTANASANA VAR. 3
(SEATED FORWARD BEND POSE, VAR. 3)

Using a chair in front of you, and sitting on some height, helps encourage an anterior pelvic tilt needed while moving into all forward bending. It is an act of kindness to greet flexibility challenges rather than push against them in the BEING variations of classic poses such as this one.

How to move into Paschimottanasana, Var. 3

1. Follow the Basic pose instructions with modified prop placement.
2. Breathe and relax.

How to come out of Paschimottanasna, Var. 3

1. Follow the Basic pose instructions.

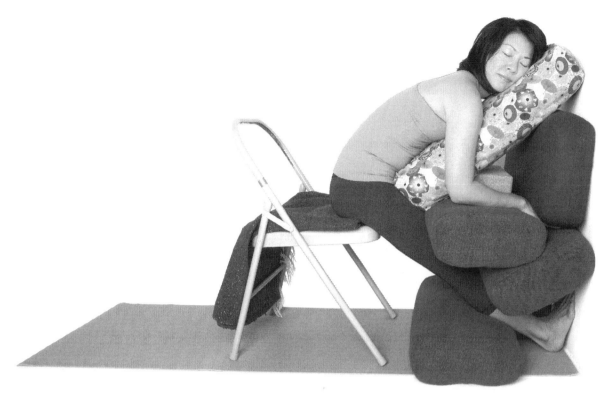

PASCHIMOTANASANA VAR. 4
(SEATED FORWARD BEND POSE, VAR. 4)

Let's say you are the student with a tight lower back and hamstrings. Perhaps you have a difficult time sitting upright without bending your knees or flexing at your lower back. This variation greatly elevates your pelvis, giving you the angle needed in order to be positioned on the front end of the buttock bones and find some length in the lower back. In addition, a bolster is placed on the floor a few inches away from the wall. The soles of the feet are positioned against the wall and the calves against the bolster. Once in the forward bend, the support offers a generous stretch to the calves. Stack up the bolsters so they meet you without loosing the length in the lower back.

If you determine that getting a safe stretch in the hamstrings is what's needed, over the deep relaxation benefits from having the head lower, this is a safe and logical variation.

How to move into Paschimottanasana, Var. 4

1. Follow the Basic pose instructions with modified prop placement.
2. Breathe and relax.

How to come out of Paschimottanasna, Var. 4

1. Follow the Basic pose instructions.

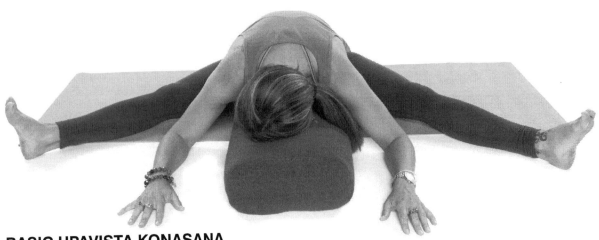

BASIC UPAVISTA KONASANA
(BASIC SEATED WIDE ANGLE POSE)

Do you wonder why you are challenged in a seated forward bend when the legs are together, but less so when they are apart? Easy, it's your hamstrings. The hamstrings are made up of two muscles (semitendinosus and semimembranosus) that run medially, or on the inner side of the thighbone, and one muscle (biceps femoris) that runs laterally, or on the outer side of the thighbone. When the legs are closer together the lateral hamstrings receive the greatest stretch. When the legs are further apart, the medial hamstrings receive the greatest stretch.

Most people have imbalances where the medial muscles are loser or shorter than the lateral muscles and vice versa. Therefore, you may find that your forward bend with legs close together is more challenging than when you separate your legs. Also, separating your legs may give you a little more room in your hips to move into a better neutral starting pelvic position. Each of these variations meets several levels of flexibility. Each of these variations meets several levels of flexibility.

How to move into Basic Upavista Konasana

1. Sit down with the legs stretched out to the sides close to 90°.
2. Place the short end of a bolster against the pelvis and belly.
3. Stretch the arms overhead and lengthen the waist, grow long, and sit up taller.
4. Stretch forward to rest the torso and head on top of the bolster, turning the head in one direction.
5. Keep your hips releasing into the floor.
6. Relax and breathe.

How to come out of Basic Upavista Konasana

1. Lift out of the pose either with a flat back or rolling out vertebrae by vertebrae.
2. Pause.
3. Prepare for what's next.

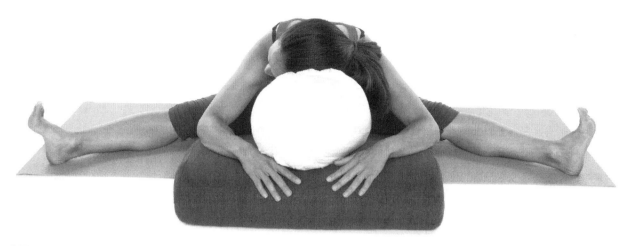

UPAVISTA KONASANA, VAR. 1
(SEATED WIDE ANGLE POSE, VAR. 1)

A simple modification like this one uses two bolsters stacked in a "T" with the arms loosely draped over the bottom bolster. Bring the top bolster all the way up against the pelvis and belly for total support. It's that easy.

How to move into Upavista Konasana, Var. 1

1. Follow the Basic pose instructions with modified prop placement.
2. Breathe and relax.

How to come out of Upavista Konasana, Var. 1

1. Follow the Basic pose instructions.

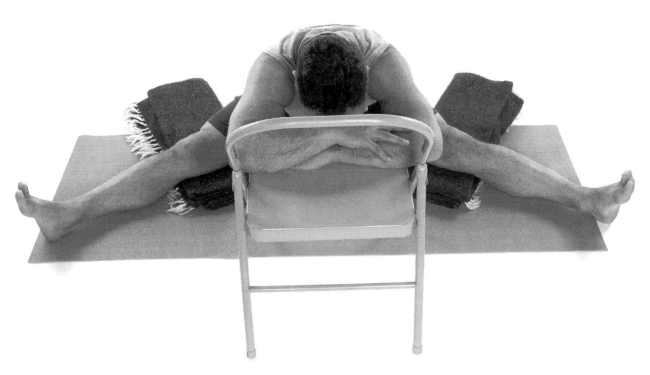

UPAVISTA KONASANA, VAR. 2
(SEATED WIDE ANGLE POSE, VAR. 2)

If you need considerable support underneath your pelvis to sit upright easily, it may put quite a bit of daylight between the backs of the legs and the floor. In this variation the legs are supported so they are not hovering above without feedback underneath them to relax. If you are better at hinging forward with a lot of support underneath your hips, you are probably the candidate who also does better with the height of a chair for your arm support. You'll be giving up the cushioned support of a bolster being right up against you, but you will be maintaining the important Hip Hinge skill for safe alignment.

How to move into Upavista Konasana, Var. 2

1. Follow the Basic pose instructions with modified prop placement.
2. Breathe and relax.

How to come out of Upavista Konasana, Var. 2

1. Follow the Basic pose instructions.

The right prop support can teach a skill necessary for experiencing a balanced approach for doing, being and breathing in a yoga pose.

CHAPTER 7
OTHER POSE OPTIONS

The following poses consist of those that are practiced seated, supine (on your back), prone (on your belly), and side lying. The seated and side lying poses stretch the sides of the body. The supine and prone poses are considered "hip openers" as they stretch the legs and hips, with the exception of one shoulder stretch on your back.

SEATED

General Contraindications

- Knee injury
- Hamstring injury
- Groin injury

General Benefits

- Stimulates abdominal organs
- Improves digestion

BASIC PARIVRTTA JANU SIRSASANA
(BASIC REVOLVED HEAD TO KNEE POSE)

This is a challenging pose for many. That's why practicing with support makes it accessible for most. The only way to stretch the front, back, and side waists at the same time is to practice a side bend and this always involves stretching an arm overhead and flexing at the waist. The quadratus lumborum, an important postural muscle that rests deep in the back waist, receives a tremendous stretch here. With the exception of a few standing and seated poses, and Balasana (Child Pose) variations, no other pose targets it like a side bend. If you sit for prolonged periods of time, this muscle can get very short and tight.

The challenge (and magic) of this pose is balancing the side stretch and gentle rotation of the chest without lifting the pelvis off the floor. Consider placing a blanket underneath the seat to help maintain a neutral pelvic position. When the head reaches the chair it should be in the same general plane as the chest rather than falling off the top of the spine, or struggling to meet the height of the chair. If this is the case, you can build up the seat of the chair with more blankets, but you risk loosing the length in the waist. If that happens, raise the chair on blocks so you are working with the appropriate height of the chair based on the height of your body.

There may be a tendency to "work" this pose. Refrain from doing so. Once you find the right support it will encourage your "heart space" to shine and any heaviness to melt away.

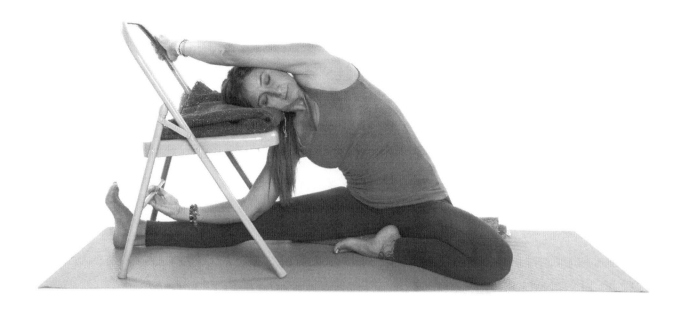

How to move into Basic Parivrtta Janu Sirsasana

1. At one end of the mat, position a sturdy chair with a folded blanket on top.
2. Stretch the right leg through the bottom frame of the chair and bring the left foot in toward the pelvis like in Baddha Konasana (Bound Angle Pose), and consider placing a meditation pad underneath the left buttock if it is hovering.
3. Hold onto the bottom run of the chair with the right hand.
4. Lengthen the waist before stretching the left arm overhead to reach for the farthest chair-back.
5. Rest the head on the blanket and turn the chest toward the sky.
6. Relax and breathe.

How to come out of Basic Parivrtta Janu Sirsasana

1. Release both hands to stretch up and into an upright position.
2. Pause.
3. Prepare for the opposite side.

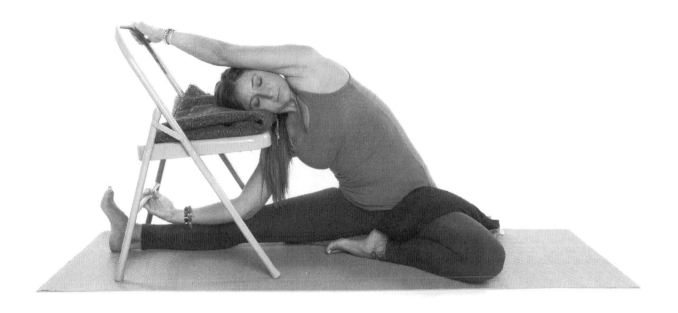

PARIVRTTA JANU SIRSASANA VAR. 1
(REVOLVED HEAD TO KNEE POSE, VAR. 1)

If stretching the top arm proves difficult, reduce the reach by holding onto any part of the chair-back. "Grounding" the bent leg is always an option and actually helps to stretch the side body even more and assists the top arm in its role to stretch and reach.

How to move into Parivrtta Janu Sirsasana, Var. 1

1. Follow the Basic ose instructions with modified prop placement.
2. Breathe and relax.

How to come out of Parivrtta Janu Sirsasana. Var. 1

1. Follow the Basic pose instructions.

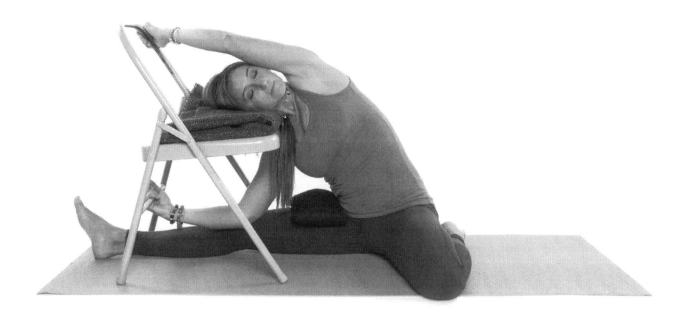

PARIVRTTA JANU SIRSASANA VAR. 2
(REVOLVED HEAD TO KNEE POSE, VAR. 2)

If the hamstrings of the straight leg need a little more flexibility support, placing a 10 lb. sandbag is an excellent option. The more flexibility coming from the straight leg, the better access to a safe hip hinge in this pose. Also, you can adjust the bent leg into another position like Virasnaa (Hero Pose) as shown below. Ask yourself what you need and why?

How to move into Parivrtta Janu Sirsasana, Var. 2

1. Follow the Basic pose instructions.

How to come out of Parivrtta Janu Sirsasana, Var. 2

1. Follow the Basic pose instructions.

SIDE LYING

General Contraindications

- Serious back injury – consult a qualified yoga therapist
- Serious shoulder injury – modify placement of bottom arm

General Benefits

- Relieves mild backaches
- Improves ribcage mobility

SIDE LYING STRETCH POSE

This is a mini variation of Parvitta Janu Sirsasana (Revolved Head to Knee Pose) without the work in the legs. The BEING versions of this pose are excellent opportunities to passively attend to muscle tightness on all sides of the waist and rib cage. Let the stretch percolate over time. Like in many other poses, the head should be supported in the same plane as the chest so it is not dropping off the top of the spine or pushed above it.

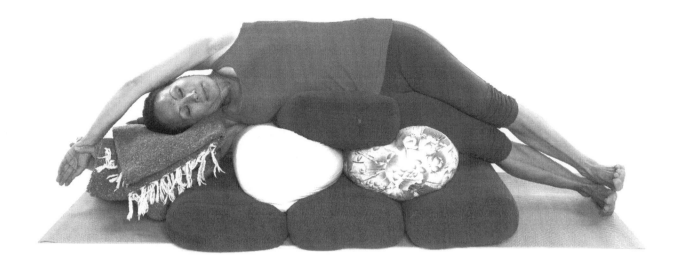

BASIC SIDE LYING STRECH POSE

How to move into Basic Side Lying Stretch Pose

1. Prepare the bolster support like in Basic Viparita Dandasana
   (Two Legged Inverted Staff Pose), pg. 56
2. Lean the right side onto the support and place a folded blanket between
   the bottom arm and the head.
3. Stretch the right arm, so the side waists are well stretched.
4. Stretch the left arm overhead, using the right hand to take hold of the wrist.
5. Straighten the legs and rest the head on the blanket.
6. Breathe and relax.

How to come out of Basic Side Lying Stretch Pose

1. Release the top arm and rest it at the top hip.
2. Bend the knees.
3. Lean the chest toward the support and use the hands to push up and sit back
   into a comfortable position.
4. Pause.
5. Prepare for the opposite side.

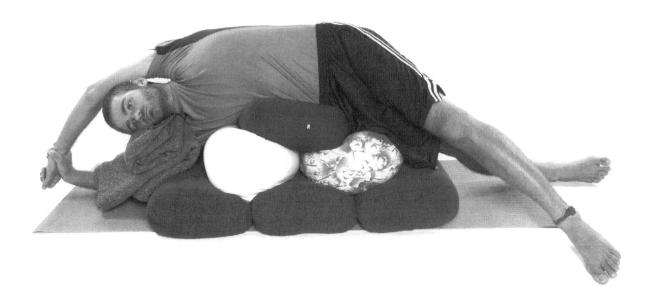

SIDE LYING STRETCH POSE, VAR. 1

Simply changing the legs into a "scissor kick" position, where the top leg stretch forward of the bottom leg, can provide a stretch to the illiotibial band (IT band), a large tendon that runs along the outer legs. A tight IT band can result in knee pain, as part of its job is to stabilize the outer knee joint. Runners, walkers, and cyclists may benefit from this variation, as this tendon is easily overused in these activities.

How to move into Side Lying Stretch Pose, Var. 1

1. Follow the Basic pose instructions with modified prop placement.
2. Breathe and relax.

How to come out of Side Lying Stretch Pose, Var. 1

1. Follow the Basic pose instructions.

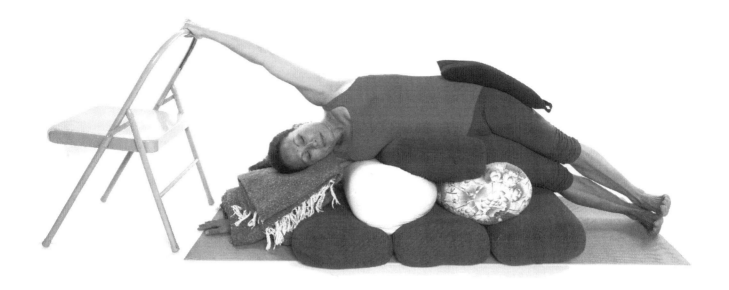

SIDE LYING STRETCH POSE, VAR. 2

Less is more. Does the top arm have a difficult time reaching overhead without rounding the shoulders or back? Of course there are a myriad or reasons for shoulder inflexibility. But, because this is also a side-bending pose, the latisimus dorsi (lateral back muscles) may be the culprit. If they are tight, they limit the range of motion in the shoulders. Modify the height of the support for the top arm as much as necessary and that includes keeping the top arm out of the stretch all together. Doing so, however, will lessen the side stretch. Choose wisely.

How to move into Side Lying Stretch Pose, Var. 2

1. Follow the Basic pose instructions with modified prop placement.
2. Breathe and relax.

How to come out of Side Lying Stretch Pose, Var. 2

1. Follow the Basic pose instructions.

SUPINE STANDING

Supine standing pose variations offer a unique opportunity to stretch areas that may be bypassed as a result of being upright. They provide a wonderful way to understand personal alignment without being in a weight-bearing position.

General Contraindications

- SI Joint Dysfunction – consult a qualified yoga therapist
- Hamstring injury
- Groin injury

General Benefits

- Improves digestion
- Helps to alleviate general back pain

BASIC SUPTA TRIKONASANA (BASIC RECLINING EXTENDED TRIANGLE POSE)

Extended Triangle on the floor -- prepare for a delicious stretch! The wall and the floor provide excellent feedback for finding a neutral pelvis. If you get confused, just imagine that your feet are standing on the floor and you are in the classic upright position.

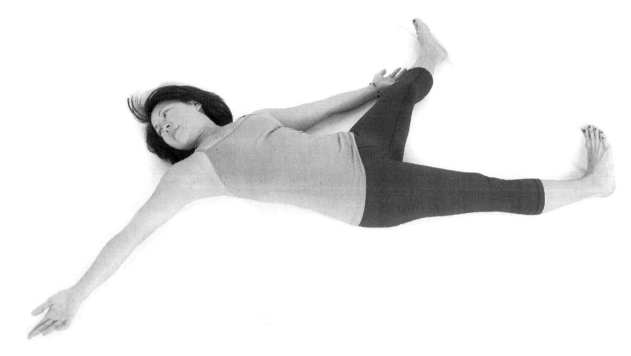

BASIC SUPTA UTTHITA TRIKONASANA
(BASIC EXTENDED TRIANGLE POSE)

How to move into Basic Supta Uttihita Trikonasana

1. Lie down on the ground near a wall and position the feet where the floor and wall meet approximately 3-1/2 to 4-1/2 feet apart, rotating the right foot out 90° and turning the left foot in about 15°.
2. Gently push your legs away from your center, and stretch your arms out into a "T" position.
3. Lengthen your waist, hinge at the front hip and slide your torso and right arm to the right.
4. When you cannot extend flex any farther, lower your right hand to the front leg and reach your left arm out with the palm facing upward.
5. Either turn the head over the left arm or keep in a neutral position.
6. Breathe and relax.

How to come out of Basic Supta Utthita Trikonasana

1. Bend the back knee and place the foot on the floor.
2. Draw the left arm into the chest.
3. Roll to the right side.
4. Pause.
5. Prepare for the opposite side.

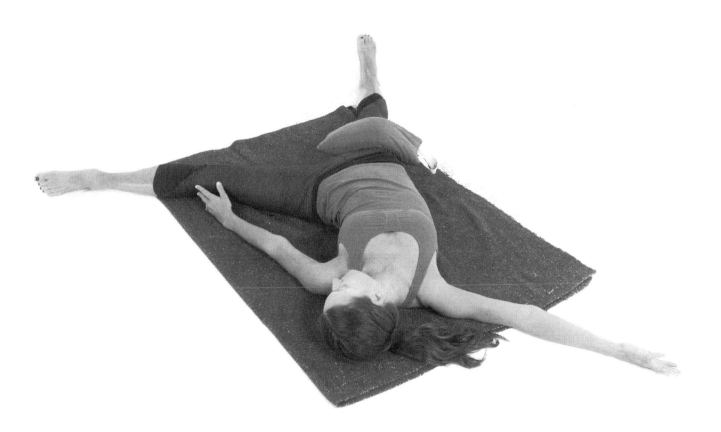

SUPTA UTTHITA TRIKONASANA VAR. 1
(RECLINING EXTENDED TRIANGLE POSE, VAR. 1)

When practiced upright, if the back collapses it may be a sign of either poor muscle flexibility or weakness. Using a 10 lb. sandbag on top of the back thigh addresses the flexibility issue by slowly increasing the stretch of that leg. The added weight helps to keep the mid buttock on the ground, which promotes an even stretch across the front of the hips.

How to move into Supta Utthita Trikonasana, Var. 1

1. Follow the Basic pose instructions with modified prop placement.
2. Breathe and relax.

How to come out of Supta Utthita Trikonasana, Var. 1

1. Follow the Basic pose instructions.

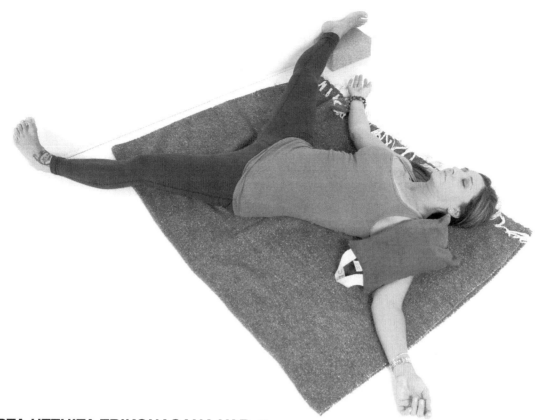

SUPTA UTTHITA TRIKONASANA VAR. 2
(RECLINING EXTENDED TRIANGLE POSE, VAR. 2)

Both of the shoulders in the pose should remain on the floor so there is an equal stretch across the front of the chest and the shoulders themselves. In this variation, a 10 lb. sandbag is placed across the far shoulder, which, due to the pose's trajectory, is the one that receives the greatest stretch. Also, the front foot is shown elevated. It keeps weight equally distributed on both mid buttocks and keeps the stretch from loading in the knee.

How to move into Supta Utthita Trikonasana, Var. 2

1. Follow the Basic pose instructions with modified prop placement.
2. Breathe and relax.

How to come out of Supta Utthita Trikonasana, Var. 2

1. Follow the Basic pose instructions.

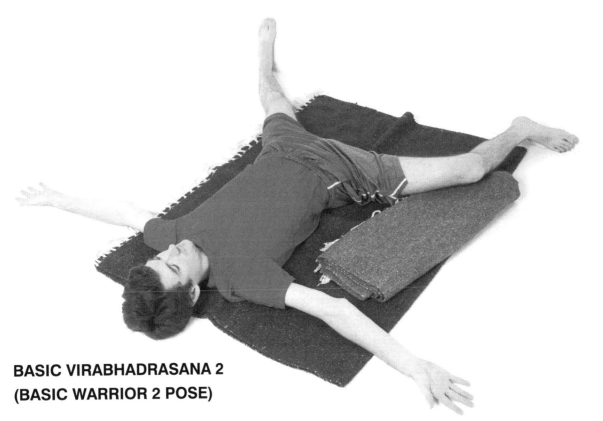

BASIC VIRABHADRASANA 2
(BASIC WARRIOR 2 POSE)

Similar to Supta Utthita Trikonasana, this pose stretches the front of the pelvis, hips, and legs and both mid buttocks should remain on the floor. If the bent leg is hovering more than an inch or two off the floor, place support underneath it so the muscles can receive feedback to relax.

How to move into Basic Supta Virabhadrasana 2

1. Lie down on the ground near a wall and position the feet where the floor and wall meet approximately 3-1/2 to 4-1/2 feet apart, rotating the right foot out 90° and turning the left foot in about 15°.
2. Bend the right leg into a 90° angle and slide closer to the wall if necessary to find proper alignment.
3. Stretch the arms into a "T" position with the palms turned upward.
4. Drop the front ribs.
5. Either turn the head to look over the right arm or keep in a neutral position.
6. Breathe and relax.

How to come out of Basic Supta Virabhadrasana 2

1. Bend the back knee and place the foot on the floor.
2. Draw the left arm into the chest.
3. Roll to the right side.
4. Pause.
5. Prepare for the opposite side.

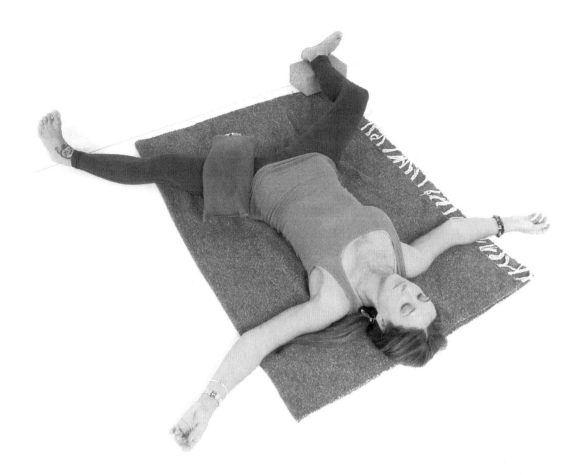

SUPTA VIRABHADRASANA 2, VAR. 1
(WARRIOR 2 POSE, VAR. 1)

Typically, in this pose if the knee of the bent leg is higher than the hip line, the foot should be elevated. Otherwise, the weight of gravity will settle in the front hip and eventually load unequally in the lower back. A 10 lb. sandbag is placed on the back leg to help weight it.

How to move into Supta Virabhadrasana 2, Var. 1

1. Follow the Basic pose instructions with modified prop placement.
2. Breathe and relax.

How to come out of Supta Virabhadrasana 2, Var. 1

1. Follow the Basic pose instructions.

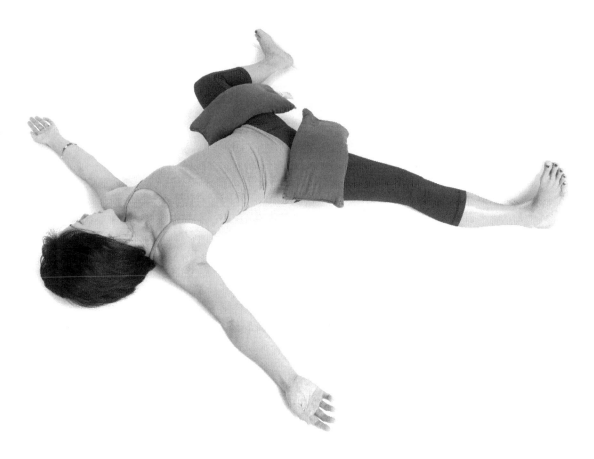

SUPTA VIRABHADRASANA 2, VAR. 2 (WARRIOR 2, VAR. 2)

For the ultimate passive "hip opener," try a sandbag on each thigh. The only candidates for this are those who can easily keep the knee of the bent leg in the same plane as the hip. Basically, the front knee should not be hovering above ground. Once this is achieved, the sandbags provide a welcome prop that releases the hips for a deep opening.

How to move into Supta Virabhadrasana 2, Var. 2

1. Follow the Basic pose instructions with modified prop placement.
2. Breathe and relax.

How to come out of Supta Virabhadrasana 2, Var. 2

1. Follow the Basic pose instructions.

SUPINE FOR LEGS

General Contraindications

- Hamstring injury
- Groin injury

General Benefits

- Improves digestion
- Relieves backaches
- Good for menstrual cramps

LEG STRETCHING SERIES
BASIC ARDHA APANASANA (BASIC HALF KNEE TO CHEST POSE)

The next several poses, the Supta Padagusthasana variations and this pose, Ardha Apanasana, can be practiced together as a therapeutic sequence for the legs and lower back. Since the health of the hamstrings in part inform the health of the lower back, each pose offers an opportunity to safely stretch the hamstrings. Besides the obvious prop support, what makes them true BEING poses is eliminating the work of the arms. There is no pulling on the belt to try and do more. Simply adjust the belt's tension to increase or decrease the stretch. Sometimes we have to actively choose to do less on our mat rather than chase the greatest sensations. With the right support, your muscles can organically stretch out during meaningful time spent in the pose. Doing so may bring a newfound approach to your practice that not only supports the life of the pose, but also fosters a deeper relationship with your practice and how you receive and perceive it.

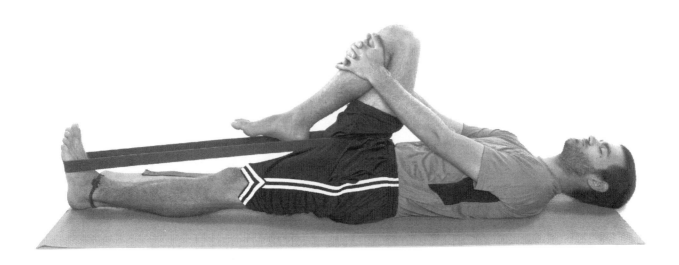

BASIC ARDHA APANASANA
(BASIC HALF KNEE TO CHEST POSE)

How to move into Basic Ardha Apanasana

1. Measure a yoga belt the length of the entire leg and have nearby.
2. Lie down on your back bend and bend the right leg.
3. Place the belt around the sole of the left foot and the top thigh (near the hip crease) of the right leg.
4. Catch the upper shin with the hands and draw the leg in toward the chest.
    Be sure to adjust the belt as necessary to maintain a level of tension between the two legs.
    without hindering the flexion of the right hip and knee.
5. Stretch the tailbone toward the left foot to lengthen the lower back.
6. Breathe and relax.

How to come out of Basic Ardha Apanasana

1. Release the bent leg and set the foot on the ground.
2. Bend the opposite leg.
3. Pause.
4. Prepare for the opposite side.

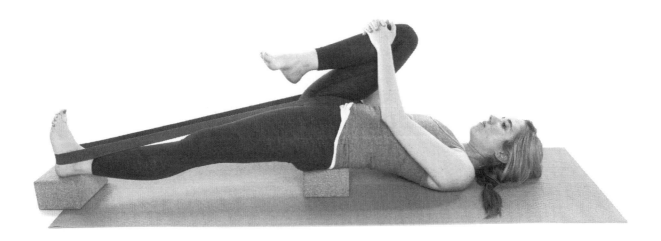

ARDHA APANASANA, VAR. 1
(HALF KNEE TO CHEST POSE, VAR. 1)

Here is an awesome way to target the hip flexors (muscles on the front side of the hip joint). Elevating the pelvis with a block changes the plane between it and the shoulders, offering a stretch to the quadriceps and hip flexors. This variation shows a block underneath the foot of the straight leg just in case the elevated pelvis creates a shortening in the lower back.

How to move into Ardha Apanasana, Var. I

1. Follow the Basic pose instructions with modified prop placement.
2. Breathe and relax.

How to come out of Ardha Apanasana, Var. 1

1. Release the bent leg and set the foot on the ground.
2. Bend the opposite leg.
3. Push the feet into the ground to lift the pelvis and slide the block out from underneath it.
4. Pause.
5. Prepare for the opposite side.

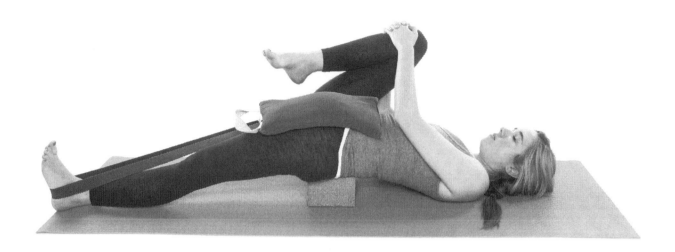

ARDHA APANASANA, VAR. 2
(HALF KNEE TO CHEST POSE, VAR. 2)

This variation takes it up a notch by eliminating the block underneath the foot of the straight leg and placing a 10 lb. sandbag on the top thigh. The combination of lowering the foot so the pelvis is the highest point in the pose, and the additional weight, offers the deepest stretch to the flexors.

How to move into Ardha Apanasana, Var. 2

1. Follow the Basic pose instructions with modified prop placement.
2. Breathe and relax.

How to come out of Ardha Apanasana, Var. 2

1. Follow the Basic pose instructions.

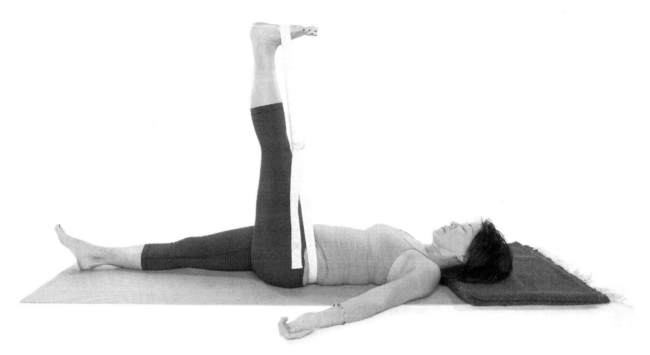

BASIC SUPTA PADAGUSTHASANA 1
(BASIC RECLINING BIG TOE POSE 1)

Like Ardha Apanasana (Half Head to Knee Pose) this BEING pose creates traction
and balances both sides of the lower back. The floor is the perfect feedback for how the
hamstrings play a role in the position of the pelvis. When you stretch the leg up to the
ceiling, notice how the pelvis moves either forward or backward the closer you bring the
leg to the torso. Keep the leg straight while maintaining a neutral pelvic position. The belt
is placed at the lower back to stabilize the stretch by drawing the leg into the pelvis.

How to move into Basic Supta Padagusthasana 1

1. Measure a yoga belt the length of the entire leg and have nearby.
2. Lie supine on the floor with the knees bent.
3. Place the belt around the lower back and the left sole of the foot and
    extend the leg to the ceiling.
4. Stretch the right leg out in front of you.
5. Relax the arms alongside the body with the palms turned upward.
6. Breathe and relax.

How to come out of Basic Supta Padagusthasana 1

1. Bend the top leg, hug the knee into the chest a few moments, and then
    place the foot on the floor.
2. Bend the bottom leg and place the foot on the floor.
3. Pause.
4. Prepare for the opposite side.

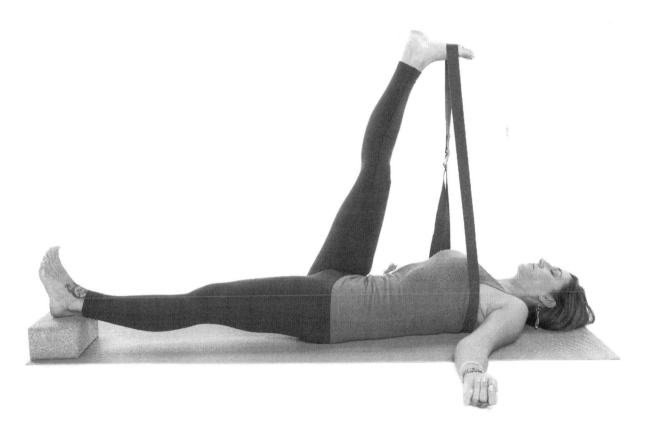

SUPTA PADAGUSTHASANA, 1, VAR. 1
(RECLINING BIG TOE POSE 1, VAR. 1)

If the leg that's perpendicular can stretch beyond a 90° position, then slide the belt up to the mid/upper back. The angle will provide a stronger pull on the leg, but if the leg naturally stretches beyond the 90°, then the hamstrings can handle it. You always have the option to place a block underneath the foot of the lower leg to avoid any pull on lower back.

How to move into Supta Padagusthasana 1, Var. 1

1. Follow the Basic pose instructions with modified prop placement.
2. Breathe and relax.

How to come out of Supta Padagusthasana 1, Var. 1

1. Follow the Basic pose instructions.

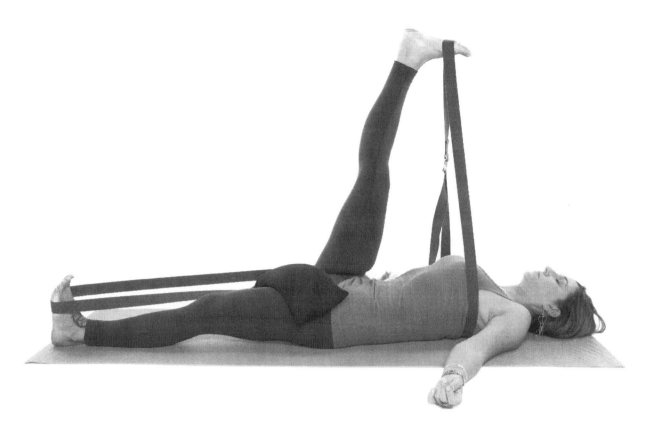

SUPTA PADAGUSTHASANA 1, VAR. 2
(RECLINING BIG TOE POSE 1, VAR. 2)

This variation is very supportive to hamstring and hip flexor flexibility and of all the variations, providing the most amount of traction to the lower back. The additional belt around the foot of the lower leg and the thigh of the upper leg gives the perfect feedback to foster lower back relief from a decompressed spine.

How to move into Supta Padagusthasana 1, Var. 2

1. Follow the Basic pose instructions with modified prop placement.
2. Breathe and relax.
3. Prepare for the opposite side.

How to come out of Basic Supta Padagusthasana 1, Var. 2

1. Follow the Basic pose instructions.

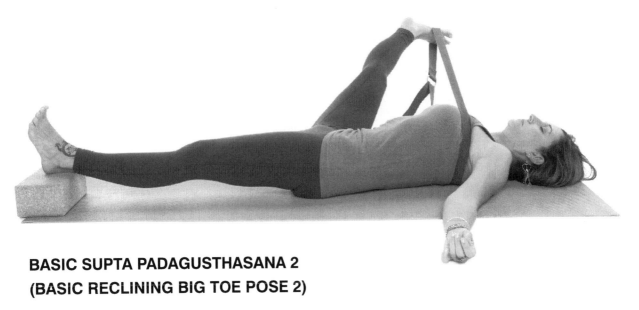

BASIC SUPTA PADAGUSTHASANA 2
(BASIC RECLINING BIG TOE POSE 2)

This pose begins in Basic Supta Padagusthasana 1 and then rotates the perpendicular leg out to the side. There may be a tendency to throw the leg out as if it is disconnected from the body's center. Instead, while you are moving the leg out, consider ways in which your movement integrates the stretch into your center rather than pull away from it. If the BEING poses are adequately supported you can spend more than just five or ten breathes in them. They are not meant to take you to your physical edge from the get go. I'm not saying you aren't going to feel sensations or that you shouldn't. I'm saying that if you practice moving in and out of these poses including this one, with an interest to generate sukha (happy/good space), you will be in balance with what this style of practice is teaching.

You can use support for the leg to rest against or not. The belt is positioned how it was in Supta Padagusthasana 1, Var. 2 (Reclining Big Toe Pose 1, Var. 2). And a block is underneath the foot of the leg that's on the floor to manage the level of stretch to the lower back.

How to move into Basic Supta Padagusthasana 2
1. Place a double-folded blanket or bolster to the right of the mat.
2. From Basic Supta Padagusthasana 1 (Basic Reclining Big Toe Pose 1), turn the right thighbone out (external rotation) while simultaneously stretching it to the right to rest the upper leg onto the support.

How to come out of Basic Supta Padagusthasana 2

1. Stretch the leg back into Basic Supta Padagusthasana 1 (Basic Reclining Big Toe Pose 1).
2. Bend the top leg, hug the knee into the chest a few moments, and then place the foot on the floor.
3. Bend the bottom leg and place the foot on the floor.
4. Pause.
5. Prepare for the opposite side.

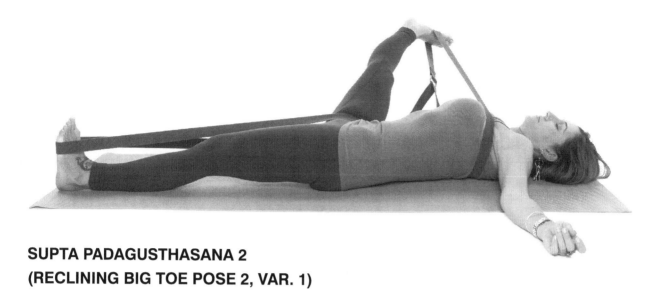

SUPTA PADAGUSTHASANA 2
(RECLINING BIG TOE POSE 2, VAR. 1)

This variation is set-up just like Supta Padagusthasana 1, Var. 2 (Reclining Big Toe Pose 1, Var. 2). It provides a lot of feedback and support. The lower belt provides excellent feedback for maintaining external rotation of the leg and a neutral pelvis, while the upper belt supports the stretch of the leg as it is being drawn into the center.

How to move into Supta Padagusthasana 2, Var. 1

1. Follow the Basic pose instructions with modified prop placement.
2. Breathe and relax.

How to come out of Supta Padagusthasana 2, Var. 1

1. Follow the Basic pose instructions.

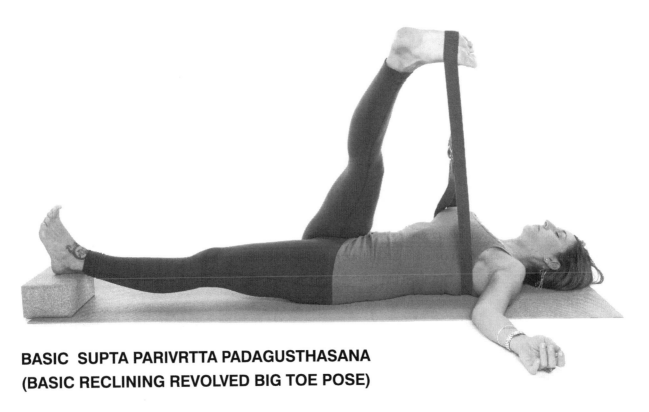

BASIC SUPTA PARIVRTTA PADAGUSTHASANA
(BASIC RECLINING REVOLVED BIG TOE POSE)

This sequence began by stretching the front of the legs, followed by the back, inner, and now finishing with the outer legs. These poses may be practiced individually or in the series. This pose offers an opportunity to stretch the largest skeletal muscle in the body, the gluteus maximus (buttocks). It's not important how close you can get the stretched leg to the floor. The value in this pose is keeping to the alignment of both sides of the lower back remaining in contact with the floor without being too rigid as your body responds to the movement of the breath and the changes in the stretch.

How to move into Basic Supta Parivrtta Padagusthasana

1. From Basic Supta Padagusthasana 1 (Basic Reclining Big Toe Pose 1), turn the right thighbone out (external rotation) while simultaneously stretching it across the torso to the left.

How to come out of Basic Supta Parivrtta Padagusthasana

1. Stretch the leg back into Basic Supta Padagusthasana 1 (Basic Reclining Big Toe Pose 1).
2. Bend the top leg, hug the knee into the chest a few moments, and then place the foot on the floor.
3. Bend the bottom leg and place the foot on the floor.
4. Pause.
5. Prepare for the opposite side.

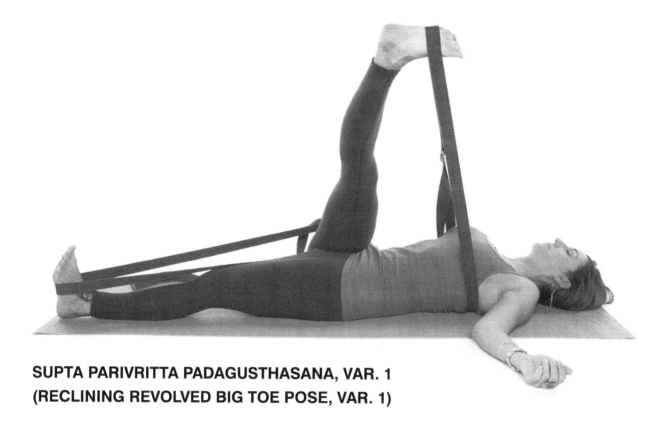

SUPTA PARIVRITTA PADAGUSTHASANA, VAR. 1
(RECLINING REVOLVED BIG TOE POSE, VAR. 1)

Do you see the pattern? Each variation of this series offers the exact set-up that provides necessary feedback and support to stretch the legs, stabilize the pelvis, and keep safe alignment.

How to move into Supta Parivrtta Padagusthasana, Var. 1

1. Follow the Basic pose instructions with modified prop placement.
2. Breathe and relax.

How to come out of Supta Parivrtta Padagusthasana, Var. 1

1. Follow the Basic pose instructions.

SUPINE FOR SHOULDERS

General Contraindications

- Shoulder injury

General Benefits

- Improves shoulder mobility and flexibility

- Improves mid and upper back mobility

- Relives upper back and neck tension

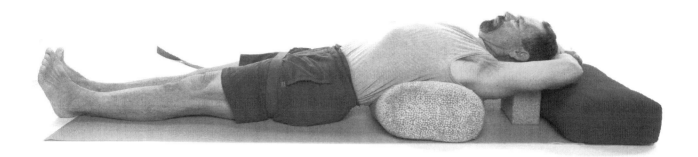

RECLINING SHOULDER STRETCH

A superb way to open the mid back and stretch the shoulders. The bolster is placed across the shoulder blades, a block for the head to rest on, and another bolster to catch the weight of the folded arms. Awesome!

How to move into Reclining Shoulder Stretch

1. Position two bolsters and a block across your mat; one bolster at the top end and the other approximately 8" away with the block on its flat, wide side in between.
2. Stretch your legs out and fasten a yoga belt firmly around the top thighs.
3. Sit in front of the bottom bolster approximately 6" away.
4. Place the hands on the floor on either side of your hips and while lifting the chest, lie back until the shoulder blades touch the top of the bolster and the head rests on the block.
5. Stretch your arms overhead, then bend the arms and cradle an elbow in each hand. Reverse your elbow hold halfway through.
6. Breathe and relax.

How to come out of Reclining Shoulder Stretch

1. Release the arms from overhead.
2. Bend the knees and place the feet on the floor.
3. Draw the left arm in to your chest.
4. Push off the feet and roll to the right.
5. Pause.
6. Prepare for what's next.

PRONE POSES

Prone poses are atypical in that in all pose classifications, there aren't a lot of poses that are practiced face down. Here is another example of strategic prop placement in order to provide ample support for the most amount of comfort. Positioning the body face down is required in all prone poses and may bring attention to stiffness and tension of which you are unaware. Just remember to breathe into what is happening now, and be ever mindful of SAS to prevent over-stretching or misalignment.

General Contraindications

- Ankle injury
- Knee injury
- Groin injury
- SI Joint Dysfunction

General Benefits

- Blood flow to pelvic organs
- Lower back relief
- Improves hip flexion flexibility

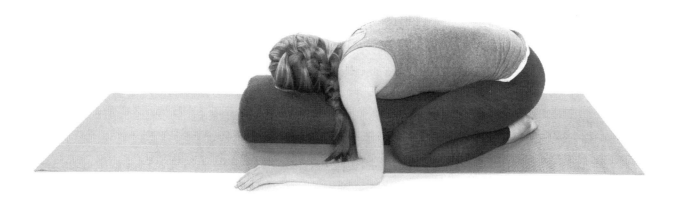

BASIC BALASANA (BASIC CHILD POSE)

Generally, this pose is loved by all with the exception of those whose hips and or knees cannot or should not hyper flex. It is the perfect pose to practice after a twist as it settles the back into a neutral position, which is important after rotating the spine. It provides welcome relief for those with a tight lower back. There is one rule that should be followed: The shoulders and hips are to be kept in the same plane – neither one should be above or below the other. This ensures that the pose is achieving a balance of flexibility between of hip flexion and lower back.

How to move into Basic Balasana

1. Start in a table position on hands and knees, resting on the tops of the feet.
2. Position the legs wide enough to rest outside of your side ribs, and slide a bolster between the legs.
3. Bend at the hips to bring the pelvis down to the heel bones while resting the torso on the bolster.
4. Turn the head to the right so the right nostril is on top.
5. Rest the arms in a goal post position.

How to come out of Basic Balasana

1. Keep the chin in a neutral position relative to a neutral skull.
2. Turn the head to rest the forehead on the bolster.
3. Place the hands on the floor underneath the shoulders and straighten the arms to lift the torso away from the bolster.
4. Sit back on the heels or in any comfortable position.
5. Pause.
6. Prepare for what's next.

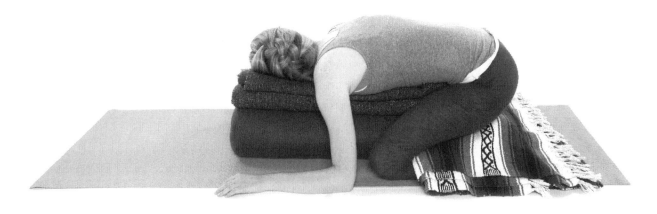

BALASANA VAR. 1 (CHILD POSE, VAR. 1)

Here is how you bring the pose to those who don't have the shoulders and hips in the same plane. Build the support up enough until this is achieved. If building up the torso support means that the hips still hover over the heels, consider placing a blanket between the legs and the hips. This is also a good option for someone who requires less flexion in the knees. When using support for this purpose, place the long folded edge of the blanket all the way into the knee crease. And if the elbows hover and are no longer in the same plane as the hands, then fill that space with support, too.

How to move into Balasana, Var. 1

1. Follow the Basic pose instructions with modified prop placement.
2. Breathe and relax.

How to come out of Balasana, Var. 1

1. Follow the Basic pose instructions.

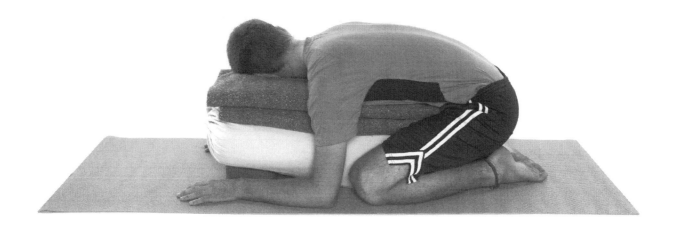

BALASANA VAR. 2 (CHILD POSE, VAR. 2)

Another way to bring the pose to the student is to elevate the top end of the support, bringing a slight angle as shown here. I've added a few more double-folded blankets to fill the space between the body and support. This is a good option if the hips are releasing, but the torso still drops below the hip line.

How to move into Balasana, Var. 2

1. Follow the Basic pose instructions with modified prop placement.
2. Breathe and relax.

How to come out of Balasana, Var. 2

1. Follow the Basic pose instructions.

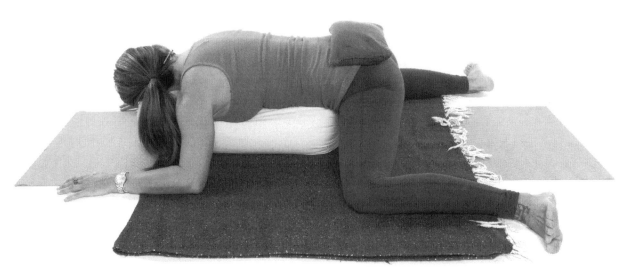

BASIC BHEKASANA (BASIC FROG POSE)

You either love to love this pose, or love to avoid it. This pose offers a generous stretch to the adductors (inner thigh muscles), which are also considered balancing agents for our legs. We need them strong and flexible in order to walk and balance without falling over. Similar to Balasana (Child Pose), position the support to keep the shoulders and hips in same plane when possible. Never overstretch. If the weight ends up loading a collapsed lower back or a dipped chest, keep exploring a better set-up. Finding the right support may take some time, but is well worth the effort and patience.

How to move into Basic Bhekasana

1. Place a bolster parallel on the mat.
2. Start in a table position on hands and knees over the bolster.
3. Separate the legs and bring them into a 90° position so the thighs are parallel and shins are perpendicular to the floor.
4. Rest the torso on the bolster, allowing the pelvis to hang off of it, and place the arms in a goal position.
5. Turn the head to the right, so the right nostril is up.
6. Breathe and relax.

How to come out of Basic Bhekasana

1. Turn the toes in toward the tailbone.
2. Push the hands against the floor to pull your body forward and straighten the legs.
3. Bend the knees and roll to one side.
4. Pause.
5. Prepare for what's next.

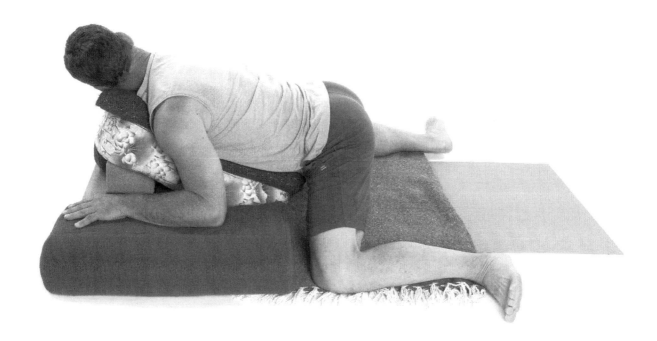

BHEKASANA VAR. 1 (FROG POSE, VAR. 1)

Here's an example of truly bringing the pose to the student. The adductors shouldn't be screaming. And you may find that even with the smartest of support, the student is still uncomfortable. Perhaps it is the general architecture of the pose, or a vulnerability that begins to surface. If a steady breath and calm mind cannot be maintained, this pose can be done on the back with the soles of the feet against the wall. Your body will be in the same shape as the pose, but on your back.

How to move into Bhekasana, Var. 1

1. Follow the Basic pose instructions with modified prop placement.
2. Breathe and relax.

How to come out of Bhekasana, Var. 1

1. Turn the toes in toward the tailbone.
2. Push the hands against the floor to straighten the arms, lifting away from the support.
3. Walk the knees behind you and then sit back into a comfortable position.
4. Pause.
5. Prepare for what's next.

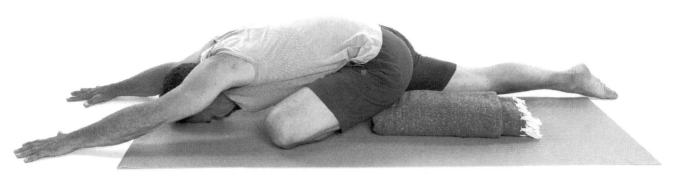

BASIC EKA PADA KAPOTASANA (BASIC ONE LEGGED PIGEON POSE)

Practicing this pose with support underneath the pelvis can increase the stretch as it lifts the pelvis, which squares itself to the front edge of the mat. This way the body doesn't tilt. If the body tilts to one side while holding the pose, the load may collect around the front knee – not what we want here! The femur (thigh bone) of the front leg must externally rotate and the external rotator muscles must have the flexibility to support the stretch to prevent any load and/or torque on the knee. This pose isn't for everyone. It can always be practiced on the back in a "figure four" stretch, which is much less risky. If equal flexibility and stability is present in the hip joint, however, it is a pose worth practicing in a prone position. Be ever vigil of your needs. Refrain from feeding your ego. It's not worth it.

How to move into Basic Eka Pada Kapotasana (Basic One Legged Pigeon Pose)

1. Position a blanket or bolster across the middle of the mat.
2. Kneel just behind the support with your hands slightly ahead of it, and step your right foot over the support.
3. Turn the right thighbone out and wiggle the right foot toward the left hand while settling the pelvis onto the support.
4. Slowly slide your left leg back, reaching all the way back to straighten the knee and drop the front of the thigh on the floor.
5. Stretch the arms forward and rest your head on the floor, or fold your arms to rest the forehead on the top arm.
6. Breathe and relax.

How to come out of Basic Eka Pada Kapotasana

1. Walk the hands closer to the support.
2. Push the hands into the floor and turn the back toes under.
3. Lift the left knee off the mat, so you can slide the support out from underneath the pelvis and roll to the right.
4. Pause.
5. Prepare for the opposite side.

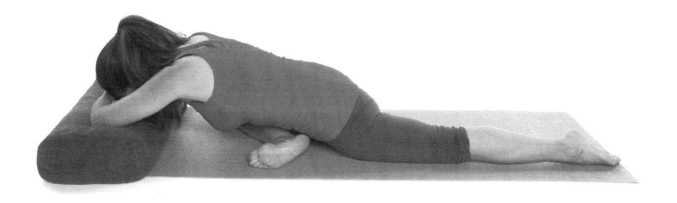

EKA PADA KAPOTASANA VAR. 1 (ONE LEGGED PIGEON POSE, VAR. 1)

This variation reduces the reach of the torso. Once the torso moves below the plane of the hips, it offers a tremendous stretch to the gluteus (buttocks) and neighboring hip muscles. A bolster or even two bolsters to catch the torso can be enough support to keep you in the pose longer than five breaths. Smile!

How to move into Eka Pada Kapotasana, Var. 1

1. Follow the Basic pose instructions with modified prop placement.
2. Breathe and relax.

How to come out of Eka Pada Kapotasana, Var. 1

1. Follow the Basic pose instructions.

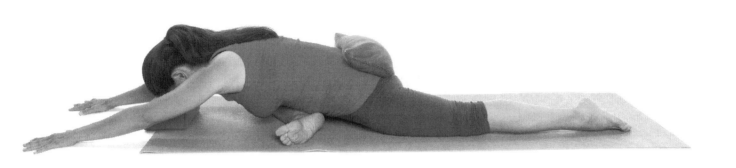

EKA PADA KAPOTASANA VAR. 2 (ONE LEGGED PIGEON POSE, VAR. 2)

If you want that extra little something, but not quite ready to stretch it all out, change out the torso support for a block at the forehead. I find this variation to be great for those who hold tension in the neck while in this pose, an indication that they aren't quite supported enough to let go. Of course, you can always add a 10 lb. sandbag across the back pelvis to encourage it to drop into gravity a little more.

How to move into Eka Pada Kapotasana, Var. 2

1. Follow the Basic pose instructions with modified prop placement.
2. Breathe and relax.
3. Drop the left knee again and roll to the right side.
4. Pause.
5. Prepare for the opposite side.

How to come out of Eka Pada Kapotasana, Var. 2

1. Follow the Basic pose instructions.

*The way our body relaxes into its Savasana shape tells us
much about challenges we may face in other poses.*

CHAPTER 8
STILL POSES:
FINAL RELAXATION THE YAPANA WAY

Savasana (Corpse Pose) is crucial to all styles of asana practices, but especially to complete a Yapana practice. Because BEING poses have prepared the body for final relaxation, to shorten or all together ignore this part of the practice would leave the student feeling incomplete. Savasana is a pose for integrating all that has come before. When we stop planning, organizing, and managing, we are able – if only momentarily – to experience the death of our doing. When this occurs, the full experience as a present moment dies, and is only a breath away. Death teaches us that time and space are temporary and that clinging to life is an aversion to change. Savasana acts as fertile ground that creates an opening for the passing and going of all that keeps us bound.

There will be times in Savasana, when you will feel "relaxation challenged." Sometimes it is because the mind is processing what has come before, or out of nowhere sensations and emotions begin to bubble to the surface. The way our body relaxes into its Savasana shape tells us much about challenges we may face in other poses, whether they require more physical effort or not. Becoming aware of our holding patterns in stillness is just as important as observing them in movement, and a pointer to what kind of support might be necessary to promote more balance overall to our body/mind when practicing Savasana.

Like in all yoga poses, there are levels of experience that change with time spent in a pose. It is not unlikely to be disturbed in Savasana, even after a complete BEING practice. However, both thoughtful and skillful sequencing of the Yapana BEING and STILL segments will encourage the most amount of rest with the least amount of effort. And allowing yourself to accept the changes of feelings and sensations, as opposite as they may appear, will foster an experience of reconciliation and integration rather than separation.

In a Yapana practice, we allow for a minimum of 15 minutes for final relaxation. Studies have shown that most people require up to 15 minutes to drop into a state of relaxation. You don't have to be bound to practicing BEING poses before Savasana. In fact, I recommend practicing Savasana every day, with or without BEING poses. Try it for seven straight days and see what comes. Savasana has strong potential for showing you a doorway into mindfully managing life and promoting feelings of expansion and joy.

How Would You Like Your Savasana?

There are many ways to take rest in Savasana, with or without support. Savasana does not have to be practiced the exact same way every time. Determining the kind of Savasana for the practice is based on what kinds of poses, or Pranayama, were practiced before Savasana. For instance, if the sequence addressed a stiff lower back, it may be a logical choice to offer a Savasana that gives support to the lower back. If this is the case, consider practicing Savasana with either the legs elevated or weight on the top thighs to release the lower back into gravity.

Or, if the sequence focused opening the chest and shoulders, it may be a logical choice to practice a Savasana that includes an eye pillow to support going inside.

Preparation for a Pranayama Practice

Perhaps you have a pranayama practice toward the end of the asana practice. If so, you may have done poses that focus on opening the front, back and side waists, muscles between the chest and shoulders. Practicing a "mini" Savasana (approximately 3 minutes) is recommended before a pranayama practice. This can help further mentally prepare for pranayama. Of course, after pranayama practice is completed, a full Savasana is recommended.

General Contraindications

- Pregnancy – after first trimester, elevate the chest so the heart is higher than the belly

General Benefits

- One-pointed awareness
- Mental clarity
- Helps to lower blood pressure
- Helps with insomnia
- Reduces fatigue
- Relaxes body
- Relieves stress

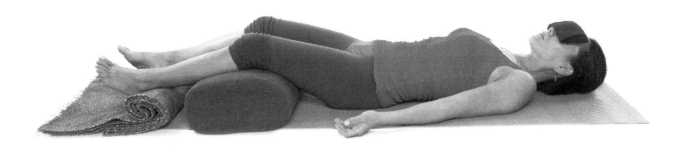

BASIC SAVASANA (BASIC CORPSE POSE)

When practicing Corpse Pose, it may take a few moments to settle into position. Move around a bit to find a good level of comfort and then commit to where you are. Allow a gentle breath to move in and out, gently rocking your body away from and into gravity.

This simplest of support is shown, a bolster and blanket to support the legs, and an eye bag to rest across the eyes.

How to move into Basic Savasana

1. Rest supine with the legs draped over a bolster and a single or double rolled blanket behind the ankles.
2. Rest the arms and hands away from the hips.
3. Make comfortable distance between the shoulders and ears.
4. Relax the skin of the forehead, eyes, and cheeks down toward the bridge of the nose.
5. Deliberately relax the weight of the bones, muscle, organs, fluids, and nerves.
6. Explore and receive the feelings and sensations as they come in and out of your awareness.
7. Feel what it feels like to relax. And relax a little more.

How to come out of Basic Savasana

1. Allow movement to stir throughout the body.
2. Bend the knees, placing the feet onto the floor.
3. Draw the knees into the chest and roll to the right.
4. Pause.
5. Prepare for what's next.

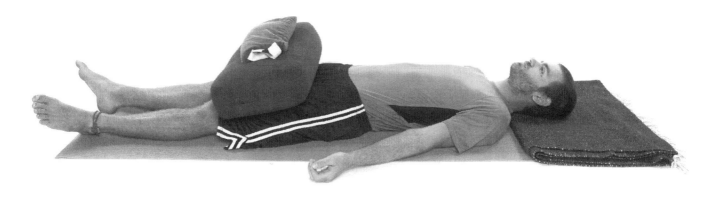

SAVASANA, VAR. 1 (CORPSE POSE, VAR. 1)

This variation uses a bolster and 10 lb. sandbag to weight down the legs and pelvis, which can bring relief to an achy or fatigued lower back.

How to move into Savasana, Var. 1

1. Follow the Basic pose instructions with modified prop placement.
2. Breathe and relax.

How to come out of Savasana, Var. 1

1. Follow the Basic pose instructions.

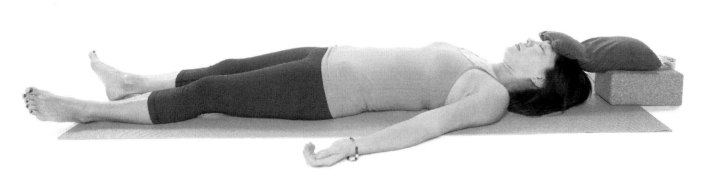

I have combined the next two variations (2 and 3) as they both address tension headaches. Although the causes of tension headaches are still uncertain, researches believe that most are triggered by internal or environmental stress. Often times the breathing pattern of someone who frequently experiences tension headaches is shallow. Or the breath is held without any awareness of doing so. Poor breathing habits influence our posture and the tension we hold in our body. Both variations aim to relax the muscles around the face, neck, throat, and shoulders.

SAVASANA, VAR. 2 (CORPSE POSE, VAR. 2)

A block is placed behind the head with a 10 lb. sandbag split into thirds. The top third of the bag is gently placed across the forehead. The weight of the bag informs the entire skull to relax into gravity.

How to move into Savasana, Var. 2

1. Follow the Basic pose instructions with modified prop placement.
2. Breathe and relax.

How to come out of Savasana, Var. 2

1. Follow the Basic pose instructions.

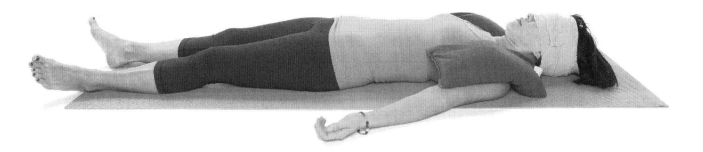

SAVASANA, VAR. 3 (CORPSE POSE, VAR. 3)

Habitual holding of the upper back and neck, and eyestrain, may trigger
tension headaches.

This variation shows an eye wrap is placed around the face to cover the forehead, ears,
and eyes. This soft compression feels comforting against the skull and acts as a quiet
cocoon refuge from the business of the external world. The sandbags on the shoulders
weight them down so the upper trapezius (large back muscles that extends from the base
of the skull to the lower mid-back and across the shoulder blades) and levator scaulae
(muscles that rest on the back and side of the neck) can relax, leaving the head, neck, and
shoulders to help melt away accumulated stress held there.

How to move into Savasana, Var. 3

1. Follow the Basic pose instructions with modified prop placement.
2. Breathe and relax.

How to come out of Savasana, Var. 3

1. Follow the Basic pose instructions.

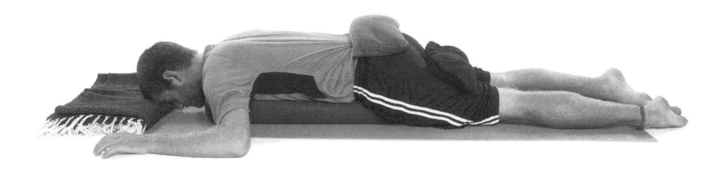

SAVASANA, VAR. 4 (CORPSE POSE, VAR. 4)

This downward facing variation of Savasana is an interesting option for someone
who may want to explore relaxation around the abdominal region. The torso is supported
on a bolster with the pubis bone water-falling off one short end of the bolster. Because
not everyone is comfortable resting on the front side of the body, a 10 lb. sandbag is
placed across the back of the pelvis and the upper back thighs to settle the pelvis into
a neutral position. If necessary, a blanket is placed underneath the head to prevent it
from falling off the top of the spine.

How to move into Savasana, Var. 4

1. Position a bolster parallel on the mat with a blanket on the floor in front of it.
2. Lie face down so the pubis bone is just hanging off the back end of the bolster.
3. Rest the forehead on the blanket.
4. Bring the arms into a goal post "T" position.
5. Relax and breathe.

How to come out of Savasana, Var. 4

1. Bend the left knee along side the bolster.
2. Push the left hand into the ground.
3. Roll to the right side.
4. Pause.
5. Prepare for what's next.

A mindfulness practice establishes an inner silence that creates a stress-free environment used to handle a stressful outer environment.

CHAPTER 9

BEING AND BREATHING: THE YAPANA WAY TO MINDFULNESS

Our world is fast paced, both internally and externally, but we do have the means to address the chaos. Science has proven that meditation sharpens the mind and produces benefits for everyone. Meditation creates change in brain waves, particularly Alpha waves, which are associated with relaxation.

Many people say they don't have the time to devote an hour a day for meditation. Each of us, however, has 10 or 15 minutes for being and breathing, which can open the door to mindfulness or a formal meditation practice. Like most things we learn, there is no way to get good at it other than doing it.

The word meditation can stir up images in our mind – from the old loin clothed yogi sitting on a mountain to a monk who has taken a vow of silence and hasn't spoken in years or a scantily clad popular yoga teacher posing on the cover of a yoga magazine. I think of meditation as practicing mindfulness and an opportunity to "be" and breathe mindfully. Mindfulness is a time to observe without judgment and take to heart what's present without pushing against or away from your self. A mindfulness practice establishes an inner silence that creates a stress-free environment used to handle a stressful outer environment.

There is no right or wrong way to meditate. It can be practiced while sitting, walking, eating, or any other time and situation you choose. For many who sit, having a comfortable seat is the biggest challenge. The following are four ways to support your "seat."

Personal freedom can be yours. You only need to make the investment – in yourself.

General Contraindications

*   None
*   Serious back injuries that should avoid long period of sitting

General Benefits

*   Mental clarity
*   Helps reduce high blood pressure
*   Helps reduce anxiety
*   Promotes feelings of steadiness and joy throughout
*   Builds self-confidence
*   Harmonizes body, mind, and spirit

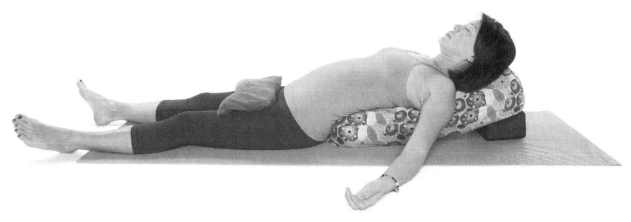

SUPPORTED RECLINING POSE

If you prefer to rest in a reclining position for mindfulness, here is a supported pose that keeps the belly, ribs, and chest open and accessible for breathing. This is considered more of a "classical" position for pranayama. It can be used for simple mindfulness practices. Or you may practice a basic breathing technique: Belly, Ribs, and Chest (see instructions below).

How to move into Supported Reclining Pose

1. Position a bolster parallel to the mat with a block underneath the top end.
2. Lie back with the small of the back against the bottom end of the bolster, resting your entire torso on the bolster.
3. Allow your arms to rest outside the hips with the palms turned upward.
4. Let the legs separate and relax.
5. If you like, place a 10 lb. sandbag on the top thighs.
6. Breathe and relax.

How to come out of Supported Reclining Pose

1. Bend the knees and set the feet on the ground.
2. Draw the left arm into the chest.
3. Push off the feet and roll to the right side.
4. Pause.
5. Prepare for what's next.

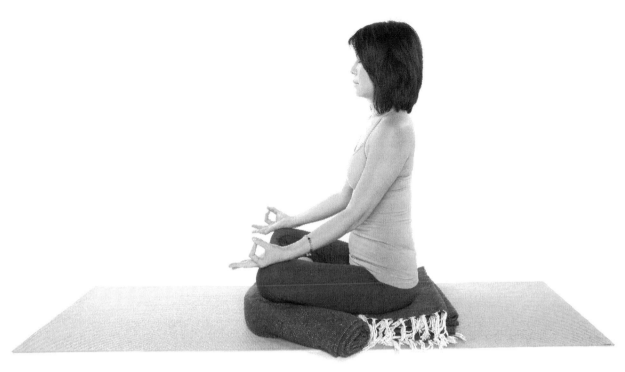

BASIC SEAT FOR MINDFULNESS

How to move into Basic Seat for Mindfulness

1. Prepare a folded meditation pad and a long-rolled blanket.
2. Sit upright near the front edge of the meditation pad in a cross-legged position.
3. Wrap the long-rolled blanket around the outer legs and allow the shins and knees to rest against it.
4. If you like, place the hands in Jnana mudra, gently touching the thumb and index fingers and lightly placing them on the tops of the knees.
5. Be with your breath.
6. Be still.

How to come out of Basic Seat for Mindfulness

1. Bring your awareness to your whole body by taking a few deep, long inhales and exhales.
2. Bring your awareness to the outer edges of your eyes.
3. When you open the eyes, allow the outer edges of the eyes to widen and the eyes themselves to relax toward the back of the sockets – let the landscape come to you rather than reaching with your sight to see it.
4. Straighten the legs.
5. Pause.
6. Prepare for what's next.

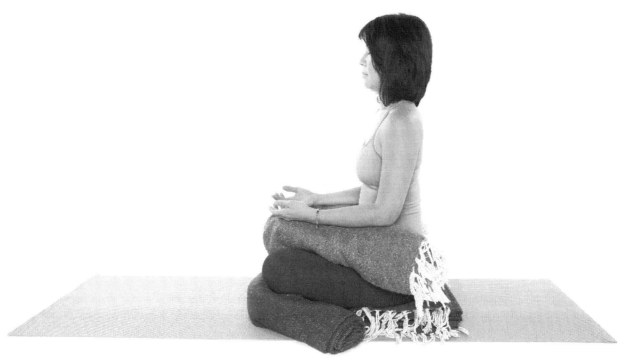

SEAT FOR MINDFULNESS, VAR. 1

This variation adds arms support. Play with the position of the hands to find out what position allows the shoulders to remain down and away from the ears and the head balanced on the top of the spine. Having the lower arms supported with double-rolled blankets underneath them provides the feedback to relax them even more.

How to move into Seat for Mindfulness, Var. 1

1. Follow the Basic pose instructions with modified prop placement.
2. Breathe and relax.

How to come out of Seat for Mindfulness, Var. 1

1. Follow the Basic pose instructions.

SEAT FOR MINDFULNESS, VAR. 2

Try this option if you prefer to sit on a chair. A belt is wrapped around the shoulders and mid back to draw the shoulders and shoulder blades back and down, and underneath the legs for lower back support. A 10 lb. sandbag is resting on the top thighs to weight down the legs, which helps to lengthen the lower back in the upright, seated position.

How to move into Seat for Mindfulness, Var. 2

1. Follow the instructions below on how to fasten the belt around your body.
2. Sit upright on the front edge of a chair with the feet hip distance apart.
3. Position the fastened belt underneath the legs and place a 10 lb. sandbag on the top of the thighs.
4. Place a 10 lb. sandbag on the top of the thighs.
5. Position the hands with the palms turned upward.
6. Be with your breath.
7. Be still.

How to fasten the belt

1. Place the yoga belt around your neck with the two tails falling equally.
2. Bring the tails underneath the armpits and behind the back.
3. Cross one tail over the other and move both tails to the front of the body.
4. Fasten the belt firmly, but it should not restrict your breathing.

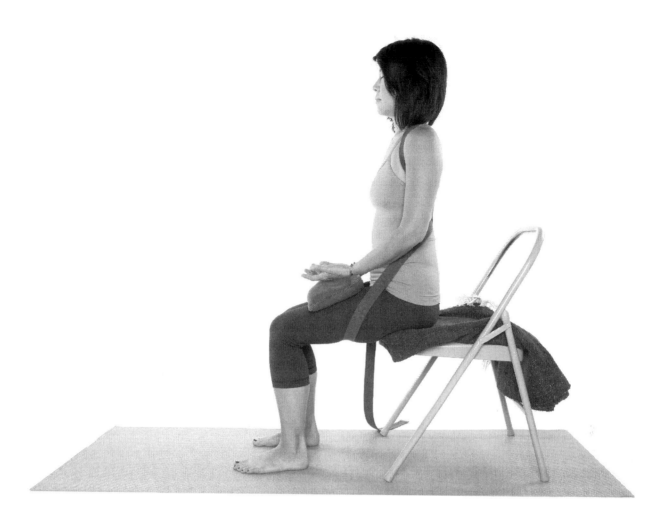

How to come out of Seat for Mindfulness, Var. 2

1. Bring your awareness to your whole body by taking a few deep, long inhales and exhales.
2. Bring your awareness to the outer edges of your eyes.
3. When you open the eyes, allow the outer edges of the eyes to widen and the eyes themselves to relax toward the back of the sockets – let the landscape come to you rather than reaching with your sight to see it.
4. Release the belt around the legs.
5. Pause.
6. Prepare for what's next.

SEAT FOR MINDFULNESS, VAR. 3

This is an excellent option for
someone who tends to collapse
in the lower and mid back. It provides
both support and feedback to the
lower and upper body including
the arms. This is one of my favorite
set-ups for my mindfulness practice.
Try it. You may love it.

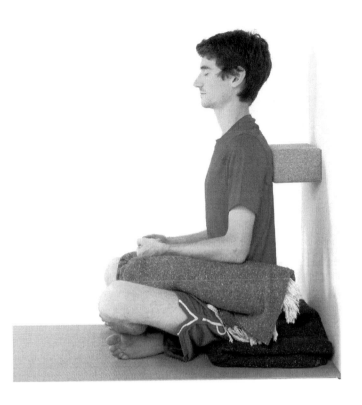

How to move into seat for Mindfulness, Var. 3

1. Position your body near a wall with a meditation pad, two short-rolled blankets, and a block.
2. Place the open-ended edge of the meditation pad next to the wall.
3. Sit upright near the front edge of the meditation pad in a cross-legged position.
4. Place the long thin side of the block between the shoulder blades and the wall.
5. Place a short-rolled blanket underneath each arm for support.
6. Use the feedback of the block to relax the shoulders, lift and broaden the chest, and align the head on top of the spine.

How to come out of Seat for Mindfulness, Var. 3

1. Bring your awareness to your whole body by taking a few deep, long inhales and exhales.
2. Bring your awareness to the outer edges of your eyes.
3. When you open the eyes, allow the outer edges of the eyes to widen and the eyes themselves to relax toward the back of the sockets -- let the landscape come to you rather than reaching with your sight to see it.
4. Reach back with a hand to remove the block.
5. Straighten the legs.
6. Pause.
7. Prepare for what's next.

THREE BASIC BREATHING (BASIC PRANAYAMA) TECHNIQUES FOR MINDFULNESS

The following breathing techniques have been around for years. They are not new and improved versions. They are an invitation for you to explore, reconcile, and accept what is present or dormant in you simply by being, breathing, and feeling. That is all. Keeping it simple is what this is all about.

BELLY, RIBS, CHEST BREATHING – 3 PART BREATHING

This is a classic introduction to exploring mindfulness via the breath and relaxes the body/mind. It is easy for yoga practitioners, once introduced to a breath called Ujjayi ("The Victorious Breath"), to be entranced with forcing the sound that it produces by making a slight closure at the root of the throat. As a result, breathing becomes strained and all sensitive observation of the breath goes out the window. Consider using this simple mindful technique, Belly, Ribs, and Chest, as a way to connect and explore what's happening now. It can be practiced as part of your BEING practice, before, or after. And it can be practiced in any of the Seats for Mindfulness or the Supported Reclining Pose.

1. Rest the hands lightly across your belly.

2. Bring your interest to the belly and feel how it gently spreads and settles from underneath your hands.

3. Breathe into a soft and merciful belly. There is no right or wrong here, except do not allow the breath to harden the belly as you bring your breath to it. Invite the breath to spread rather than lift the belly. Take your time exploring the breath and practice accepting all the feelings and sensations that may arise.

4. Slide your hands to lightly rest across the front ribs and feel how they gently expand and contract from underneath your hands.

5. Breathe into this protective structure known as the rib cage. Invite the breath to move the side and back ribs, without pushing and forcing the discovery. Take your time exploring the breath and practice accepting all of the feelings and sensations that may arise.

6. Slide your hands to lightly rest across the chest and feel how the hands may rise and fall or pull away from each other with each inhale and exhale. Explore the chest as two pieces rather than one – as if the right and left sides were two separate parts of the chest. Notice if the breath is stronger on one side than the other. There is nothing to change. Your only interest is in observation and acceptance. Take your time exploring the breath and practice accepting all the feelings and sensations that may arise.

7. Remove the hands from the chest and rest them alongside the hipswith the palms turned upward.

8. Rest.

Now combine the practice by bringing your attention to the belly and gently moving a soft, round, but deep breath up the body, into the ribs and toward the chest. Do not force this. Follow your inhale from the belly, ribs, and chest. Let a long and controlled exhale release from the belly, ribs, and chest. Pause. Take three normal paced breaths.

1. Practice several rounds without creating hardness in the belly, ribs, chest, throat, or neck.

2. When finished, observe normal paced breaths.

3. Stretch out with your feelings to sense the quality, temperature, and sensations of the breath and your overall experience of what's happening now.

4. Resist nothing, even the concept of resistance.

5. Let your body float in the sensations of its structure, support, and space.

6. When you feel ready to move, draw your interest to the solid floor beneath you.

7. Sense how your body is being moved by the movement of the breath -- away from and into gravity.

8. Allow some movement to stir throughout your body.

9. Draw your knees into the chest.

10. Pause.

11. Roll to the right side.

12. Prepare for what's next.

CENTER TO PERIPHERY BREATHING – BREATHING LIKE A BABY

This breathing technique is a balance of directing and following the breath from the navel area (we'll call that your center) and outwardly (we'll call that the periphery) to the space around you. Have you ever observed a baby breathe? The body moves gently, swaying and rocking as a result of an organic process of each phase of the breath. The Center to Periphery breathing technique gives a gentle massage to the muscles, organs and tissue that evokes an indescribable calm and steadiness throughout. Ultimately, the goal is to breathe like a baby. Practice Center to Periphery Breathing in the Reclining Supported Pose as it is easier to feel the movement of the breath against the body in a reclining position rather than a seated one.

1. Bring your awareness to your center and notice the breath gently moving you away from gravity on an inhale and settling you into gravity on an exhale.

2. Take a few breaths that are a little longer and deeper than usual to help facilitate this.

3. Now relax your skin so you can perceive the movement the breath has against it and how it plays with the force of gravity.

4. On an inhale, with the most amount of awareness and the least amount of effort, direct your breath from your center to your limbs and into the space around you.

5. On an exhale, allow the breath to release from the periphery and settle back into your center.

6. Encourage a round, global breath rather than a vertical one.

7. Follow with two or three normal paced inhales and exhales.

8. Continue again with the movement and direction of the breath.

9. When your interest has waned, return to normal paced breathing.

10. Follow the How To Come Out instructions for the Reclining Supported Pose.

EXCHANGING THOUGHTS FOR FEELINGS – BREATHING & FEELING

The BEING poses provide a safe place to introduce meditation. This breathing technique taps into the deep well of our thoughts and feelings. Exchanging thoughts for feelings is another way to extend and support the life of mindfulness. Because a thought does not want to be looked at for too long, exchanging it with a feeling is a pathway to holding awareness for a longer period of time. My personal preference is to practice this in any of the Seats for Mindfulness as sitting upright helps to keep me interested in the process.

1. Find your preferred Seat for Mindfulness.

2. Gently place your hands at your chest.

3. Start breathing mindfully.

4. Be aware of the present thought and exchange it for a feeling.

5. Be with the feeling for as long as you can until another thought wants to enter.

6. Exchange the new thought with a feeling and continue the cycle until your disinterest is stronger than your ability to hold interest.

7. To complete, take three or four deep breaths.

8. Follow the How To Come Out instructions for the Seat for Mindfulness.

There is real power in being peaceful.

CHAPTER 10
PURPOSEFUL PRACTICES

So many of us are living a disconnected life that leaves us feeling constantly busy and "stressed out." We're spending more time surviving rather than living. We've replaced a well-balanced meal with several lattes and sit in a chair in front of a computer screen for hours each day. On top of that, we have to manage all of our personal and professional obligations. This accumulation of negative energy creates a wall between our "doing" and "being" self as opposed to integrating the two. Purposeful Practices are specific sequences that help to remedy a lifestyle that overloads our system – and weakens us physically and physiologically – causing injuries, common ailments and mental and emotional trauma. Purposeful Practices provide the self-care that is necessary for shedding the stresses accumulated throughout each day.

Individual poses in a sequence can be switched out with other poses to make adjustments. However, pose placement in any sequence is important and should not be approached haphazardly. Because each pose has a physiological effect on the body/mind, their position in a sequence can alter the overall benefits of a sequence.

The following sequences are examples of what is possible. They target either specific areas of the body or common challenges. Each one is approximately 30 to 60 minutes and designed to achieve a purposeful practice for wellbeing, breakdown the wall of stress, and refuel your spiritual self. Each pose is shown in its recommended form, although you may practice any variation to meet your individual needs.

Practicing without any distractions and having access to all of your yoga props is an ideal situation. The following are recommendations to further support your journey of self-care.

- The best time to practice is when you can fully tune in and be present. Try scheduling your practice the same time of the day throughout the week to foster consistency. Whatever time you determine is best, be prepared to give yourself to it wholeheartedly.

- Turn off your phone.

- Practice in a clean and smoke-free environment that provides fresh air and is temperature controlled.

- Have all of the yoga props available and a blanket in case you get cold.

- Background music may be used to induce a state of deep relaxation.

TIME IS ON YOUR SIDE

If you are new to a supported practice, take your time here. You'll need some practice to get acquainted with positioning the yoga props so they provide the right support. Each sequence can be practiced as shown, or you can modify to meet your personal preferences. It is important, however, to consider the physiological affects that each pose provides. For instance, if you are going for total rest and relaxation, it makes less sense to practice back bends before the STILL pose because backbends are more wakeful to the nervous system, whereas forward bends and some inversions are more calming and cooling.

The following is a recommended timetable for minutes spent in poses. You can use it as a guide to help direct you into the kind of practice you wish to experience.

BEING POSES

TIMETABLE: MINUTES SPENT IN POSES	
Backbends	2-5, gradually increase to 15
Twists	3, gradually increase to 10
Forward Bends	2-5, gradually increase to 10
Inversions	3, gradually increase to 20
Lateral Bends	3, gradually increase to 5
Reclining Standing	2-5, gradually increase to 10
Reclining Leg Stretches	3, gradually increase to 5
Shoulder Stretch	3, gradually increase to 5
Prone	3, gradually increase to 5
Final Relaxation	15 - 20
Seats for Meditation	5, gradually increase to 30

Powerfully Peaceful

....

At times life can feel overwhelming. This is when we can turn to our practice to receive immediate loving care. Where practice is done, a problem is solved. A still mind is what ultimately solves a problem. This sequence is designed to still and quiet the mind and instill a calm and steadiness throughout. Practice this sequence to combat holiday stress, physical fatigue, mental exhaustion, or just plain crankiness. It you want to be at peace, you have to practice being peaceful. If you want to experience peace around you, you have to practice being peaceful. If you want others to be peaceful, you have to practice being peaceful around them.

- BELLY, RIBS, & CHEST BREATHING IN: BASIC RECLINING BOUND ANGLE POSE
- BASIC FISH POSE
- BASIC STOMACH TURN POSE
- BASIC CHILD POSE
- BASIC BRIDGE POSE
- BASIC SEATED FORWARD BEND POSE
- BASIC LEGS UP THE CHAIR POSE
- BASIC CORPSE POSE - 3 MINUTES
- EXCHANGING THOUGHTS FOR FEELINGS IN: SUPPORTED RECLINING POSE
- CORPSE POSE, VAR. 3

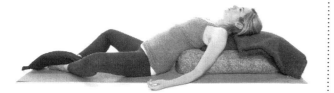

BASIC RECLINING BOUND ANGLE POSE

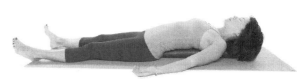

BASIC FISH POSE

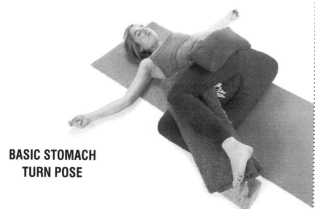

BASIC STOMACH TURN POSE

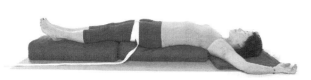

BASIC BRIDGE POSE

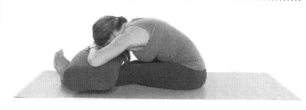

BASIC CHILD POSE

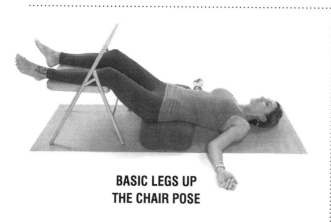

BASIC LEGS UP THE CHAIR POSE

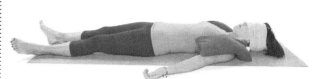

BASIC SEATED FORWARD BEND POSE

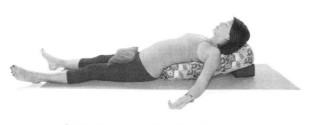

SUPPORTED RECLINING POSE

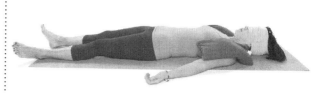

BASIC CORPSE POSE - 3 MINUTES

CORPSE POSE, VAR. 3

Stiff Shoulders

There are many factors that make up a healthy posture and the shoulders play a key roll. A slouched posture with rounded shoulders overstretch and strain the upper back and neck, and shorten and weaken the muscles between your shoulder blades. Habitual slouching collapses the chest, compresses the thoracic diaphragm, and can develop into stress injuries or dysfunction in your shoulder joints. Ouch!

This sequence focuses on releasing neck and shoulder tension while supporting and stretching neighboring muscles. It's the ultimate reversal for slouched shoulders and for someone who spends a lot of time sitting at the computer.

- RECLINING SHOULDER STRETCH
- SIDE LYING STRETCH POSE, VAR. 2
- RECLINING REVOLVED TRIANGLE POSE, VAR. 1
- BASIC CAMEL POSE
- STOMACH TURN POSE, VAR. 1
- BASIC BRIDGE POSE
- BASIC CHILD POSE
- CORPSE POSE, VAR. 3

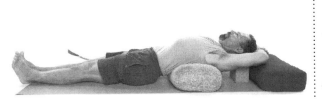

RECLINING SHOULDER STRETCH

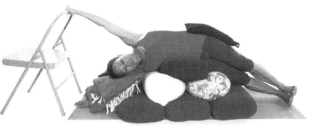

SIDE LYING STRETCH POSE, VAR. 2

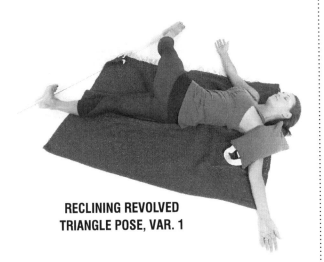

**RECLINING REVOLVED
TRIANGLE POSE, VAR. 1**

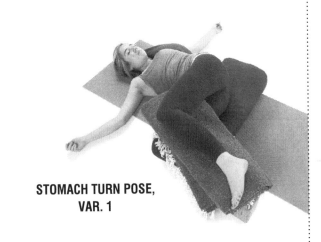

**STOMACH TURN POSE,
VAR. 1**

BASIC CAMEL POSE

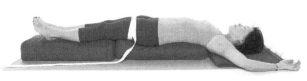

BASIC BRIDGE POSE

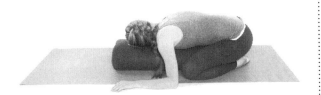

BASIC CHILD POSE

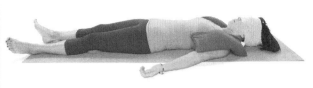

CORPSE POSE, VAR. 3

Lower Back Luck

Millions of Americans complain of lower backaches when there is nothing structurally wrong. Perhaps you strained your back lifting something, working out, or simply used poor biomechanics throughout the day to perform daily activities. Maybe you spend most of your day sitting at a computer – our bodies were not built for that. Of course, accumulated stress can settle in your back without you even knowing it.

There are several ingredients for healing an achy lower back. First, ease the mind with simple breathing exercises. Studies show that a calm approach to any physical challenge can help foster positive results. Next, determine the other ingredients are needed to promote healing. Your condition may require traction, mobility, stability, flexibility, or all of those.

This sequence encourages flexibility and traction to help eliminate tightness and compression. Follow the sequence of poses recommended and turn an achy lower back into lower back luck!

- BASIC CHILD POSE
- BASIC HALF KNEE TO CHEST POSE
- RECLINING BIG TOE POSE 1, VAR. 1
- FISH POSE, VAR. 2
- REVOLVED KNEE SQUEEZE POSE, VAR. 2
- HALF KNEE TO CHEST POSE, VAR. 1
- BASIC SEATED FORWARD BEND POSE
- BASIC LEGS UP THE CHAIR POSE
- LEGS UP THE CHAIR POSE, VAR. 1
- CORPSE POSE, VAR. 1

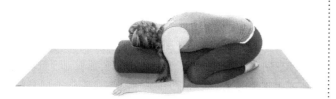

BASIC CHILD POSE

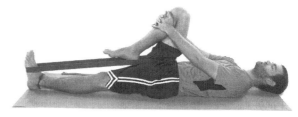

BASIC HALF KNEE TO CHEST POSE

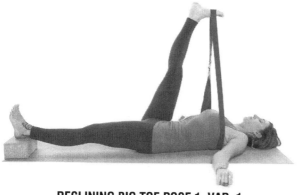

RECLINING BIG TOE POSE 1, VAR. 1

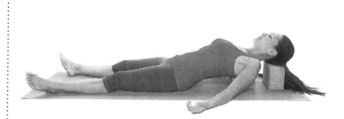

FISH POSE, VAR. 2

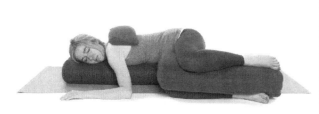

REVOLVED KNEE SQUEEZE POSE, VAR. 2

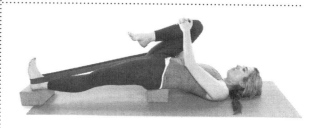

HALF KNEE TO CHEST POSE, VAR. 1

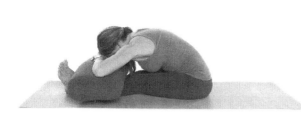

**BASIC SEATED
FORWARD BEND POSE**

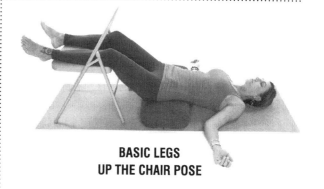

**BASIC LEGS
UP THE CHAIR POSE**

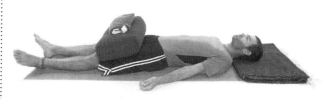

**LEGS UP THE CHAIR POSE,
VAR. 1**

CORPSE POSE, VAR. 1

Happy Hipsters

Do you need to unlock your hips? Many people have tight hip flexors (muscles that run down the front of your hip joints). Hours of sitting keep the hips in a flexed position that contracts these muscles. Hip flexors allow for forward leg movement and upward knee drive, needed in most athletics. Strategic placement of the yoga props will support the hips while gently using gravity in a friendly manner to stretch muscles and connective tissue. This sequence is comprised of seated and reclining poses and will improve your hip flexibility and mobility.

- BASIC RECLINING BOUND ANGLE POSE
- BASIC RECLINING EXTENDED TRIANGLE POSE
- RECLINING WARRIOR 2 POSE, VAR. 1
- REVOLVED HEAD TO KNEE POSE, VAR. 1
- PIGEON POSE, VAR. 2
- STOMACH TURN POSE, VAR. 2
- RECLINING BIG TOE POSE 1, VAR. 1
- BASIC RECLINING BIG TOE POSE 2
- RECLINING REVOLVED BIG TOE POSE , VAR. 1
- BASIC CHILD POSE
- BASIC LEGS UP THE CHAIR POSE
- BASIC CORPSE POSE

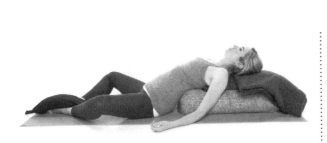

**BASIC RECLINING
BOUND ANGLE POSE**

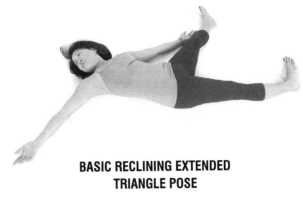

**BASIC RECLINING EXTENDED
TRIANGLE POSE**

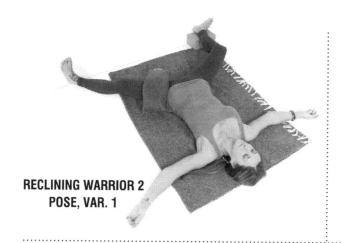

RECLINING WARRIOR 2 POSE, VAR. 1

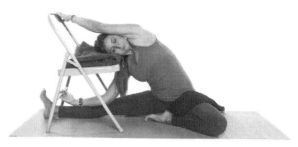

REVOLVED HEAD TO KNEE POSE, VAR. 1

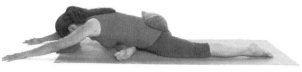

PIGEON POSE, VAR. 2

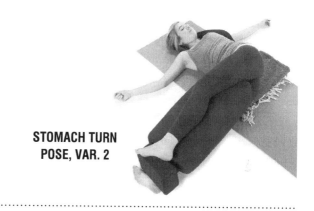

STOMACH TURN POSE, VAR. 2

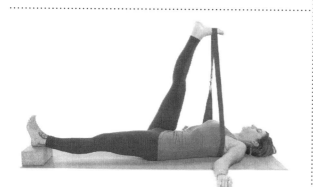

RECLINING BIG TOE POSE 1, VAR. 1

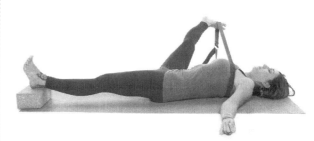

BASIC RECLINING BIG TOE POSE 2

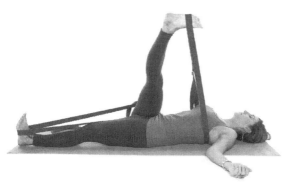

RECLINING REVOLVED BIG TOE POSE , VAR. 1

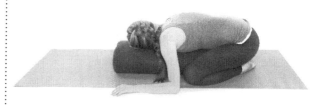

BASIC CHILD POSE

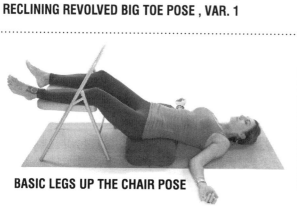

BASIC LEGS UP THE CHAIR POSE

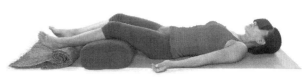

BASIC CORPSE POSE

Active Recovery for Athletes

For all the weekend warriors – this one is for you! Having worked with many professional athletes, I understand the need for active recovery from demanding workouts. Athletes may suffer from muscle soreness and imbalances by overworked muscles that can result in short and tight muscles. An intelligent Yapana BEING practice is a wise approach to repairing these muscles. The sequence focuses on stretching large muscle groups that are overloaded from repetitive movements, running, cycling, golf, and sports of all kinds.

- BASIC FISH POSE
- RECLINING BOUND ANGLE POSE, VAR. 2
- BASIC RECLINING EXTENDED TRIANGLE POSE
- BASIC RECLINING WARRIOR 2 POSE
- BASIC RECLINING REVOLVED TRIANGLE POSE
- CAMEL POSE, VAR. 2
- STOMACH TURN POSE, VAR. 1
- CHILD POSE, VAR. 1
- BASIC HALF KNEE TO CHEST POSE
- RECLINING BIG TOE POSE 1, VAR. 2
- SEATED WIDE LEGGED FORWARD BEND POSE, VAR. 2
- BASIC CORPSE POSE – 3 MINUTES
- CENTER TO PERIPHERY BREATHING IN: SUPPORTED RECLINING POSE
- BASIC CORPSE POSE

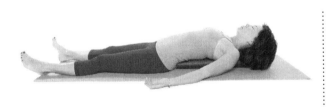

BASIC FISH POSE

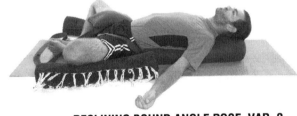

RECLINING BOUND ANGLE POSE, VAR. 2

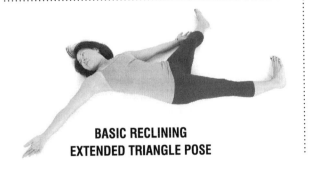

**BASIC RECLINING
EXTENDED TRIANGLE POSE**

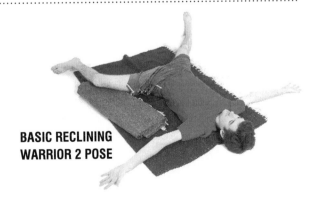

**BASIC RECLINING
WARRIOR 2 POSE**

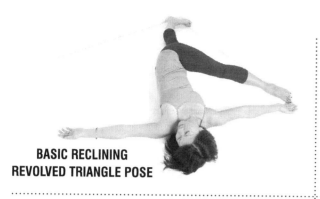

BASIC RECLINING REVOLVED TRIANGLE POSE

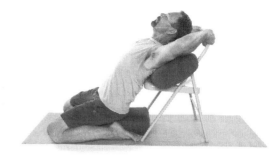

CAMEL POSE, VAR. 2

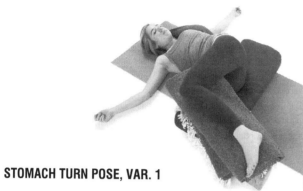

STOMACH TURN POSE, VAR. 1

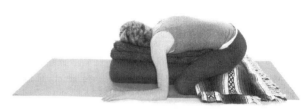

CHILD POSE, VAR. 1

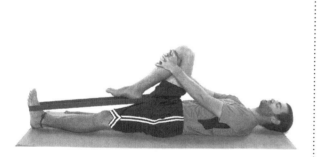

BASIC HALF KNEE TO CHEST POSE

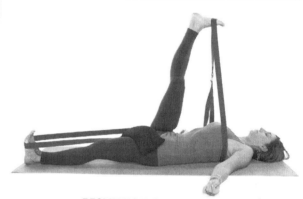

RECLINING BIG TOE POSE 1, VAR. 2

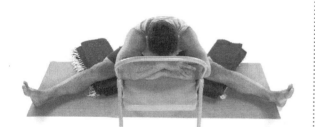

SEATED WIDE LEGGED FORWARD BEND POSE, VAR. 2

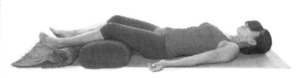

BASIC CORPSE POSE – 3 MINUTES

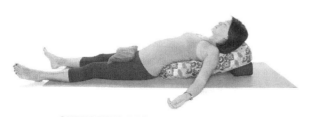

SUPPORTED RECLINING POSE

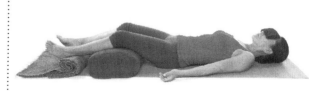

BASIC CORPSE POSE

Tension Tamer
....

Posture can effect your respiration and blood circulation to the brain, causing muscle tension that may result in a tension headache. Although a yoga practice cannot take credit for eliminating a tension headache, an intelligent Yapana BEING practice — focused on correcting poor postural habits, lengthening the neck, shoulders, and back muscles — goes a long way to reducing the potential for an impending headache caused by the shortening of these muscles.

- EXCHANGING THOUGHTS FOR FEELINGS IN: CORPSE POSE, VAR. 2
- BASIC SIDE LYING STRETCH POSE
- FISH POSE, VAR. 1
- BASIC CAMEL POSE
- BASIC REVOLVED KNEE SQUEEZE POSE
- BASIC LEGS UP THE CHAIR POSE
- BASIC BRIDGE POSE
- SEATED WIDE LEGGED FORWARD BEND POSE, VAR. 1
- BASIC SEATED FORWARD BEND POSE
- CORPSE POSE, VAR. 3

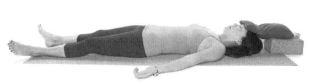

CORPSE POSE, VAR. 2

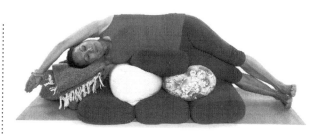

BASIC SIDE LYING STRETCH POSE

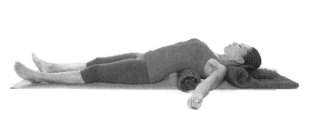

FISH POSE, VAR. 1

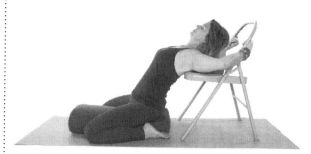

BASIC CAMEL POSE

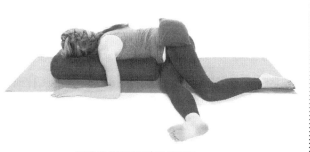

BASIC REVOLVED KNEE
SQUEEZE POSE

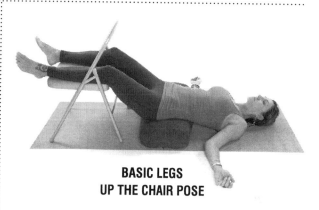

BASIC LEGS
UP THE CHAIR POSE

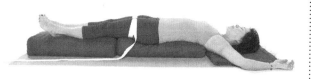

BASIC BRIDGE POSE

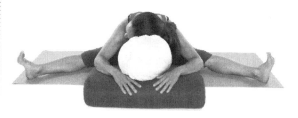

SEATED WIDE LEGGED
FORWARD BEND POSE, VAR. 1

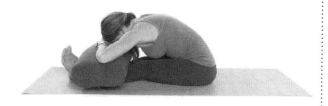

BASIC SEATED FORWARD BEND POSE

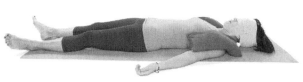

CORPSE POSE, VAR. 3

Immunity Enhancer

The adrenal glands are responsible for releasing hormones in response to stress. When the body is in constant stress mode, these glands work overtime and put strain on the immune system. This sequence focuses on preventing the adrenals from firing. I also recommend that you laugh more! Laughter stimulates circulation and aids in muscle relaxation, both of which help reduce some symptoms of stress and boost immunity. :)

- BASIC LEGS UP THE CHAIR POSE
- BASIC RECLINING BOUND ANGLE POSE
- BRIDGE POSE, VAR. 1
- BRIDGE POSE, VAR. 2
- BRIDGE POSE, VAR. 3
- BASIC FROG POSE
- REVOLVED KNEE SQUEEZE POSE, VAR. 1
- BASIC LEGS UP THE WALL POSE
- BASIC SEATED FORWARD BEND POSE
- BASIC CHILD POSE
- BASIC CORPSE POSE - 3 MINUTES
- ANY MINDFULNESS PRACTICE IN: SUPPORTED RECLINING POSE
- BASIC CORPSE POSE

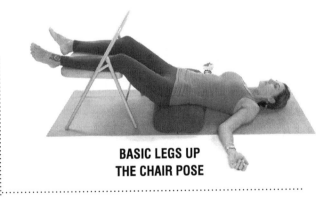

BASIC LEGS UP THE CHAIR POSE

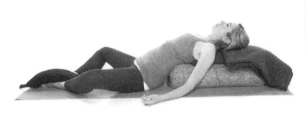

BASIC RECLINING BOUND ANGLE POSE

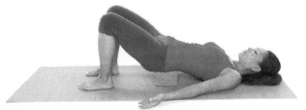

BRIDGE POSE, VAR. 1

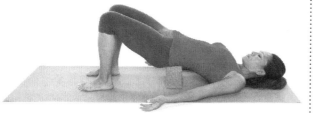

BRIDGE POSE, VAR. 2

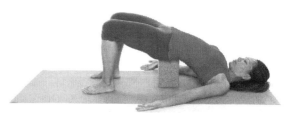

BRIDGE POSE, VAR. 3

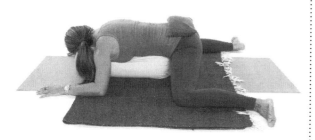

BASIC FROG POSE

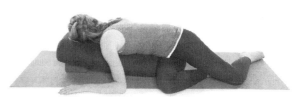

REVOLVED KNEE SQUEEZE POSE, VAR. 1

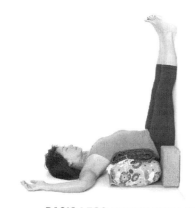

BASIC LEGS UP THE WALL POSE

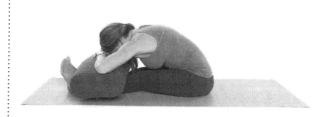

BASIC SEATED FORWARD BEND POSE

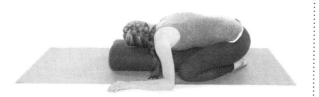

BASIC CHILD POSE

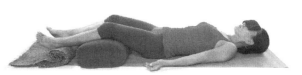

BASIC CORPSE POSE - 3 MINUTES

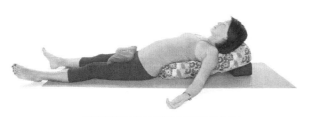

SUPPORTED RECLINING POSE

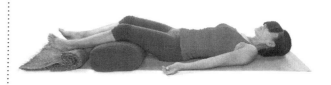

BASIC CORPSE POSE

The Women's Life Cycle

The cycles of a woman's body is both beautiful and complex. A dedicated yoga practice that includes a Yapana BEING practice supports managing the cycles with greater ease. A woman's cycles are a delicate balance of menstruation, pregnancy and menopause. The following are two Yapana BEING sequences that support two phases of the cycle. See Chapter 11 (Princess & The Pea) for a prenatal sequence.

Pelvic Wellness

The symptoms from premenstrual syndrome (PMS) include bloating, cramping, muscle tenderness, joint aches, headache, fatigue, tension, anxiety, and mood swings. Thankfully, women typically don't experience all of the symptoms listed. The Yapana BEING sequence is a complete practice that can help to decrease PMS symptoms and, in many cases, eliminate them.

- BASIC CHILD POSE
- BASIC RECLINING BOUND ANGLE POSE
- FISH POSE, VAR. 1
- BASIC RECLINING BIG TOE POSE 1
- RECLINING BIG TOE POSE 2, VAR. 1
- RECLINING REVOLVED BIG TOE POSE, VAR. 1
- SEATED WIDE LEGGED FORWARD BEND POSE, VAR. 1
- BRIDGE POSE, VAR. 1
- LEGS UP THE CHAIR POSE, VAR. 1
- BASIC CORPSE POSE

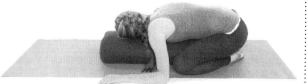

BASIC CHILD POSE

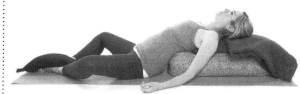

BASIC RECLINING BOUND ANGLE POSE

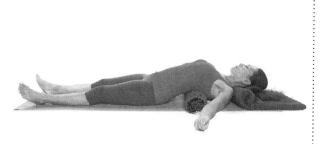

FISH POSE, VAR. 1

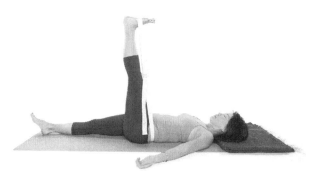

BASIC RECLINING BIG TOE POSE 1

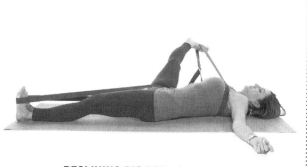

RECLINING BIG TOE POSE 2, VAR. 1

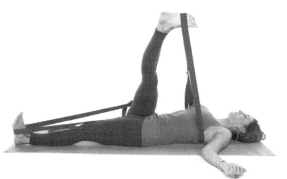

RECLINING REVOLVED BIG TOE POSE, VAR. 1

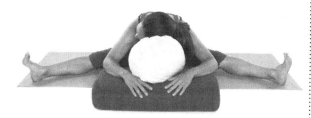

SEATED WIDE LEGGED FORWARD BEND POSE, VAR. 1

BRIDGE POSE, VAR. 1

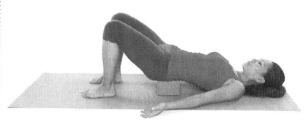

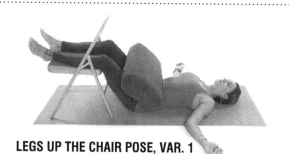

LEGS UP THE CHAIR POSE, VAR. 1

BASIC CORPSE POSE

Menopause Makeover

Menopause symptoms include hot flashes, night sweats, forgetfulness, insomnia, mood changes, weight gain, and range from irritating to debilitating. This sequence focuses on poses that help to pacify and cool the nervous system and calm your nerves. I've included one pose, Basic Inverted Staff Pose, which is the most energetic, but it is a nice opening for the back, shoulders, and front thighs and I enjoy it as part of this sequence. The practice is meant to support you. If any of the poses feel agitating, skip them. Ultimately, allow your symptoms to be a guidepost for your approach. Each day we bring a different body, mind and breath to the practice. This Yapana BEING practice promotes self-reflection and the kind of mind that quietly sits up. This level of awareness supports and directs a healthy attitude needed to face these changing times.

- BASIC LEGS UP THE WALL POSE
- BASIC RECLINING BOUND ANGLE POSE
- BASIC RECLINING EXTENDED TRIANGLE POSE
- BASIC REVOLVED HEAD TO KNEE POSE
- BASIC TWO LEGGED INVERTED STAFF POSE
- BRIDGE POSE, VAR. 1
- BRIDGE POSE, VAR. 2
- BRIDGE POSE, VAR. 3
- BASIC CHILD POSE
- BASIC SEATED FORWAR BEND POSE
- BASIC SEATED WIDE LEGGED FORWARD BEND POSE
- BASIC CORPSE POSE

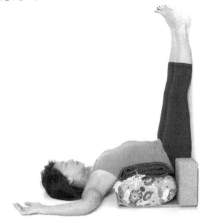

BASIC LEGS UP THE WALL POSE

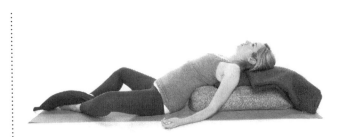

BASIC RECLINING BOUND ANGLE POSE

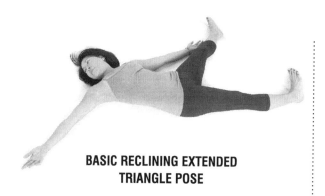

BASIC RECLINING EXTENDED TRIANGLE POSE

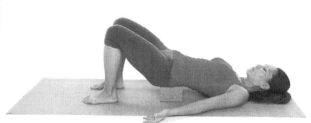

BASIC REVOLVED HEAD TO KNEE POSE

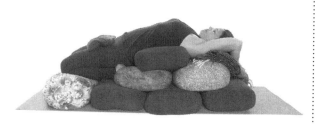

BASIC TWO LEGGED INVERTED STAFF POSE

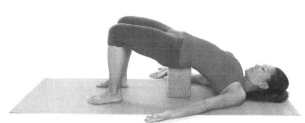

BRIDGE POSE, VAR. 1

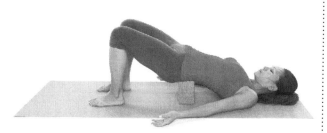

BRIDGE POSE, VAR. 2

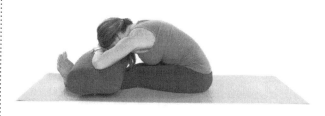

BRIDGE POSE, VAR. 3

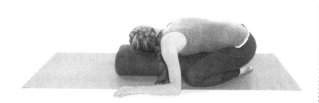

BASIC CHILD POSE

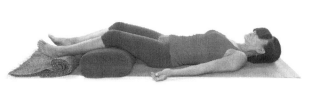

BASIC SEATED FORWAR BEND POSE

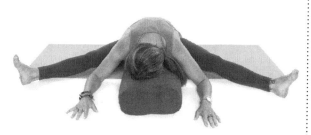

BASIC SEATED WIDE LEGGED FORWARD BEND POSE

BASIC CORPSE POSE

The right prop support can teach a skill necessary for experiencing a balanced approach for doing, being and breathing in a yoga pose.

CHAPTER 11
PRINCESS AND THE PEA

A Yapana BEING practice can serve as a healthy strategy to manage and relieve common discomforts that pregnancy may bring. It also prepares you for labor and delivery – physically, mentally, and spiritually. If you are new to a restorative yoga practice, there is no better time than at the start of your pregnancy. The gentle and therapeutic nature of this practice is the perfect combination for reducing tension and emotional stress, creating optimal health, and a positive childbirth experience for you and your baby.

Pay attention to what you feel in each pose of the sequence and, as with in any other yoga practice, trust your instincts and honor your body's needs. Western medical professionals consider the first trimester as the highest risk for miscarriage and when you experience the most changes. Be extra gentle with yourself. There is no need to push the stretches. Rather, it is relaxation that is most important. Half way, and throughout the term of your pregnancy, keep the heart higher than the pelvis in any reclining position. This ensures that the weight of your uterus doesn't compress the vena cava, a major blood vessel that is responsible for blood flow to your baby. Because the blood vessel is located to the right of your spine, some doctors recommend resting on your left side to allow blood flow more freely to your baby. Therefore, when exiting this pose, the instructions will direct you to roll to the left side. In the last trimester, consider practicing a Yapana BEING practice each day, whether it is 30 or 90 minutes. It will help to strengthen your coping mechanisms, which will come in very handy during labor! To exit the pose, you will always roll to your left.

I practiced yoga throughout all three of my pregnancies. Some days I felt like moving while other days I only wanted to practice Reclining Bound Angle Pose or Legs Up The Wall. My needs changed, as each pregnancy was different. I leaned on my practice when I needed to be held up, slowed down, or kept present. It empowered me as a woman who would be forever transformed by what was to come.

You may practice all kinds of yoga styles and make modifications to suit your growing needs. This sequence is similar to Powerfully Peaceful. Practice this Princess and the Pea sequence when you want some serious R&R and desire to deeply connect with your baby.

General Contraindications

- Like with all exercise and stretching, be sure to have your doctor's permission before continuing your yoga practice.

General Benefits

- Conscious breathing – good for managing stress levels and high blood pressure
- Stretching – keeps your body limber for the delivery
- Quiet connection with your baby

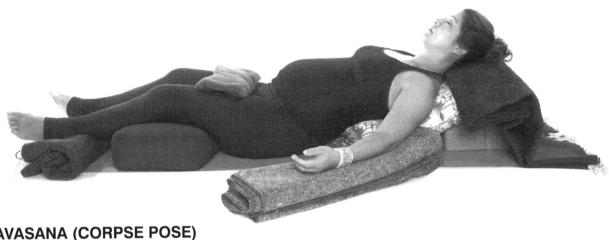

SAVASANA (CORPSE POSE)

How to move into Savasana

1. Position two bolsters on the mat; one parallel and approximately 2/3 up the top end of the mat with two blocks supported underneath the top end of the bolster, and the other bolster across the bottom end of the mat.
2. Roll a long blanket and place it at the bottom end of the mat for ankle support.
3. Place a "Foundation" or double-folded blanket across the top end of the bolster.
4. Position accordion-folded blankets on either side of the bolster to be used as arm support.
5. Have a sandbag nearby.
6. Rest supine on the bolster parallel to the mat and drape the legs over the bolster at the bottom end of the mat and the ankles on the long rolled blanket.
7. If you like, place a sandbag on the top thighs to weigh down the legs and pelvis.
8. Rest the arms and hands on the accordion folded blanket.
9. Make comfortable distance between the shoulders and ears.
10. Relax the skin of the forehead, eyes, and cheeks down toward the bridge of the nose.
11. Deliberately relax the weight of the bones, muscle, organs, fluids, and nerves.
12. Explore and receive the feelings and sensations as they come in and out of your awareness.
13. Feel what it feels like to relax. And relax a little more.

How to come out of Savasana

1. Allow movement to stir throughout the body.
2. Bend the knees, placing the feet onto the floor.
3. Draw the right arm into the chest.
4. Push the feet into the ground and roll to the left.

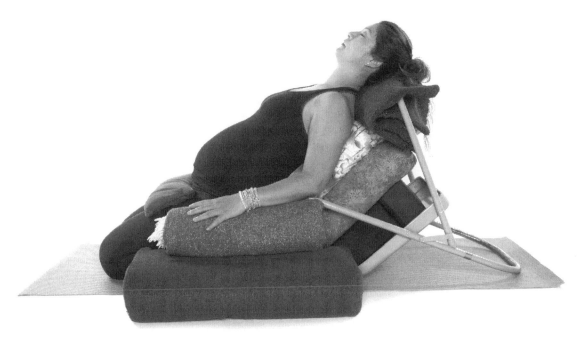

SUPTA VIRASANA (RECLINING HERO POSE)

How to move into Supta Virasana

1. Position a sturdy folding chair upside down at the top end of the mat.
2. Place two or three blocks on the underside of the chair.
3. Position two bolsters stacked length-wise on top of the blocks.
4. Cover the top back rung of the chair with a blanket.
5. Position two bolsters on either side of the chair with short-rolled blankets on top to be used for arm support.
6. Kneel in front of the support and use the hands to stretch the calf muscles away from the knees and toward the heels.
7. Place the hands on the feet to use the arms as leverage to lift the chest and safely lie back on the bolster, resting the head on the blanket and the arms on the support.
8. If you like, place a sandbag on top of the upper thighs to weight down the legs and pelvis.
9. Lift and broaden the chest.
10. Breathe and relax.

How to come out of Basic Supta Virasana

1. Gently tuck the chin.
2. Push the hands into the feet or against the floor to use as leverage to lift up and out of the pose.
3. Pause.
4. Prepare for what's next.

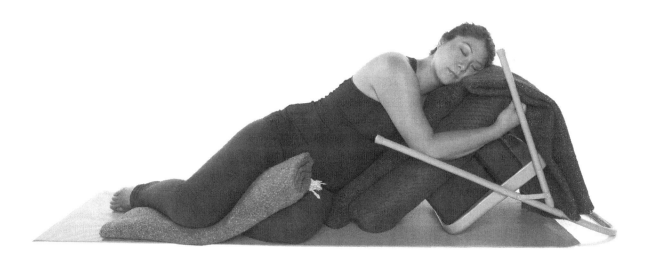

PARIVRTTA PAVANMUKTASANA (REVOLVED KNEE SQUEEZE POSE)

How to move into Parivrtta Pavanmuktasana

1. Use the same set-up as Supta Virasana, but replace the top bolster with a blanket.
2. Have a long-folded blanket available for the legs.
3. Sit the left hip against the short end of the bolster and bend both legs behind you in a soft 90° position. Place the long-folded blanket between the legs.
4. Place your hands on either side of the bolster, push them into the floor using it as leverage to lift the chest and rotate it to the left, but keep the head to the right side.
5. Lower the torso onto the bolster.
6. Place the arms in underneath the top end of the bolster.
7. Breathe and relax.

How to come out of Parivrtta Pavanmuktasana

1. Keep the chin in a neutral position relative to a neutral skull.
2. Place the hands on the floor underneath the shoulders.
3. Push the hands into the floor to straighten the arms and lift the torso away from the bolster.
4. Straighten both legs and sit upright.
5. Pause.
6. Prepare for the opposite side.

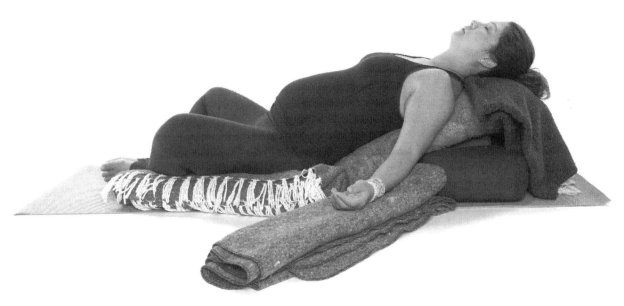

SUPTA BADDHA KONASANA (RECLINING BOUND ANGLE POSE)

How to move into Supta Baddha Konasana

1. Position a bolster parallel on your mat with two blocks supported underneath the top end of the bolster and a "Foudation" folded blanket on top of it.
2. Position accordion double-folded blankets on either side of the bolster to be used as arm support.
3. Position long-rolled blankets almost parallel to the sides of the mat to be used as leg support.
4. Sit in front of the short end of the bolster and bring the soles of the feet together so the knees and thights fall to the sides and rest on the long-rolled blankets.
5. Using your hands for support, gently lie back onto the support.
6. Allow the lower body to relax and sink into the floor and the upper body to open.
7. Breathe and relax.

How to come out of Supta Baddha Konasana

1. Gently tuck the chin.
2. Use the hands as leverage against the floor to lift up and out of the pose.
3. Slide one foot out to the side and then straighten the leg, follow by the other leg.
4. Pause with the legs straight and sit upright.
5. Prepare for what's next.

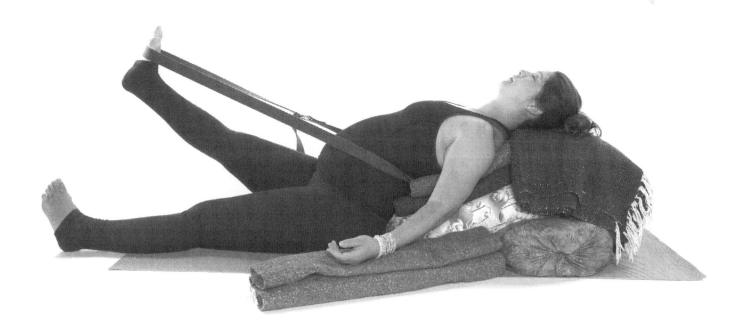

SUPTA PADAGUSTHASANA 1 (RECLINING BIG TOE POSE 1)

How to move into Basic Supta Padagusthasana 1

1. Measure a yoga belt a little longer than the length of the entire leg and have nearby.
2. Use a similar set-up similar to Supta Baddha Konasana, but replace the blocks underneath the top end of the bolster with another bolster, positioned across the mat. This will provide a little more height so the bottom bolster provides more of an angle to lift the chest.
3. Place two double-folded blankets as bolsters on top of the bolster, stair-stepped (2" distance between the bottom edges of the blankets).
4. Lie back on the bolster, place the belt around the middle back and the right sole of the foot, and extend the right leg to the ceiling.
5. Stretch the left leg out in front of you.
6. Relax the arms on the support with the palms turned upward.
7. Breathe and relax.

How to come out of Basic Supta Padagusthasana

1. Bend the right leg and place the foot on the floor.
2. Bend the bottom leg and place the foot on the floor.
3. Pause.
4. Prepare for the opposite side.
5. When both legs have been stretched, bend the knees keeping the feet as wide as the mat, and use the hands against the floor to push and sit upright.
6. Pause.
7. Prepare for the opposite side.

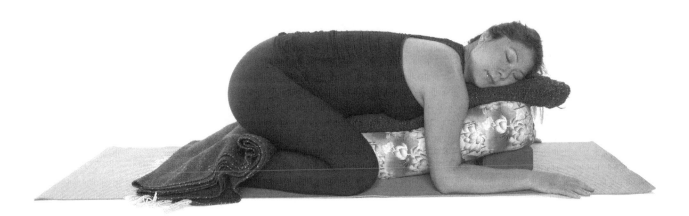

BALASANA (CHILD POSE)

How to move into Balasana

1. Start in a table position on hands and knees, resting on the tops of the feet.
2. Position the legs wide enough to rest outside of your side ribs, and slide a bolster between the legs.
3. Bend at the hips to bring the pelvis down to the heel bones while resting the torso on the bolster.
4. Turn the head to the right so the right nostril is on top.
5. Rest the arms in a goal post position.
6. If the hips do not reach the heels, place a double-folded blanket between the hips and heels to fill the space.

How to come out of Balasana

1. Keep the chin in a neutral position relative to a neutral skull.
2. Turn the head to rest the forehead on the bolster.
3. Place the hands on the floor underneath the shoulders and straighten the arms to lift the torso away from the bolster.
4. Sit back on the heels or in any comfortable position.
5. Pause.
6. Prepare for what's next.

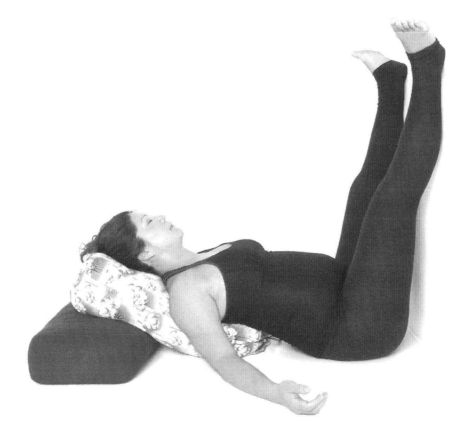

VIPARITA KARANI (LEGS UP THE WALL POSE)

How to move into Viparita Karani

1. Position two bolsters near a wall, the first bolster approximately 2' away from a wall and the other bolster underneath the top end of the bolster so the bolsters form a "T" shape.
2. Lie down against the bolster with the pelvis near the wall and the legs up the wall.
3. Bring your arms alongside the hips with the palms turned upward.
4. Breathe and relax.

How to come out of Viparita Karani

1. Bend the knees, pushing the feet against the wall. Lift the hips and shift and drop to the right.
2. Draw the right arm into the chest.
3. Roll to the left.
4. Pause.
5. Prepare for what's next.

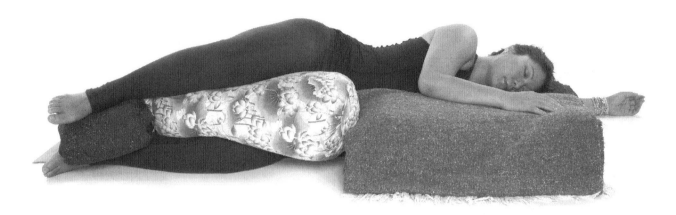

SIDE LYING SAVASANA (SIDE LYING CORPSE POSE)

How to move into Side Lying Savasana

1. Position two bolsters parallel on the mat, like a bed.
2. Place another blanket if needed, on top of the bolster closest to the head. This is needed if the elbow of the top arm needs to be more in the same plane as the shoulder.
3. Rest on the left side of the body with the top arm overhead and a blanket folded in a meditation pad placed between the arm and head.
4. Place the second bolster between the legs and place a double-folded blanket folded in half and rolled between the ankles and feet to fill the space.
5. Rest the top arm on the top bolster.
6. Breathe and relax.

How to come out of Side Lying Savasana

1. Allow movement to stir throughout the body.
2 Push into the right hand and lift the body to an upright position.
3. Pause.
4. Prepare for what's next.

The light of wisdom that lives within us is so powerful
it can turn winter into spring.

CHAPTER 12
OUR PRACTICE NEVER ENDS

Life presents abundant opportunities to return to our practice over and over. We all experience challenge and success, heartache and joy. Falling back on unhealthy habits keeps us trapped in our smaller selves and distances us from deeply taking charge of our self-care and wellbeing.

The Yapana BEING and STILL poses transform the way we see, experience, and accept things in ourselves, in others, and in the world around us. Yapana practice provides insight into the kind of mind and attitude needed for living a balanced life on and off the yoga mat.

Our practice offers us time to work hard and time to be soothed. The Yapana BEING and STILL segments cultivate a relaxed body, quiet mind, and soothes our soul.

Our practice is now. Now. And now.

Namaste.

With gratitude, I stand on the shoulders of all my teachers.
They have shared with me an abundance of knowledge and experience that has
inspired me to explore and share the path of yoga with others.

About Leeann Carey

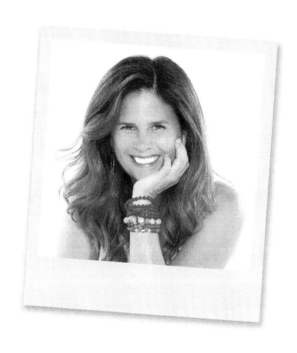

Leeann fell in love with yoga in the late 1970s, and has never wavered in her passion to share the transformational benefits of this ancient yet timeless science of life. Leeann shares that knowledge today through Yapana restorative yoga therapy teacher training programs and workshops, and through LCY mentors across the United States and Canada.

In 1993, Leeann opened the first full-service yoga studio in her South Bay community of Southern California. There she developed important skills for operating a successful "yoga business" and went on to create a teacher training school and the Yapana restorative yoga therapy program. Her eclectic blend of yoga appeals to a wide range of students and was forged over many years of study with gifted teachers including Kofi Busia, Donna Farhi, Richard C. Miller, Erich Schiffmann, and Judith Lasater.

An ERYT-500 certified instructor, Leeann has mastered the traditional techniques and developed new approaches to serve and support any student – young or old, fit or physically challenged – to enrich their lives in body, mind, and spirit. She has applied her knowledge and experience to help professional athletes, including the World Champion Los Angeles Lakers and Olympic Gold Medal Volleyball player Eric Fonoimoana, heal from injuries and improve their workouts and sports performance.

For more information on Yapana practice, teacher training and events, visit LeeannCareyYoga.com.

POSE INDEX

U

V

13537484R00117

Made in the USA
San Bernardino, CA
25 July 2014